Deconstructing the OSCE

D1589326

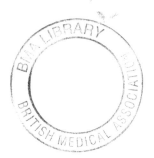

WITHDRAWN FROM

BRITISH MEDICAL ASSOCIATION

0822122

Deconstructing the OSCE

Duncan Harding PhD MRCPsych

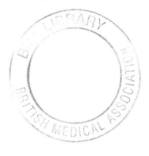

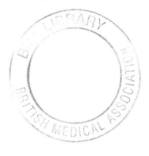

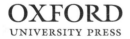

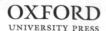

OXFORD
UNIVERSITY PRESS

Great Clarendon Street, Oxford, OX2 6DP,
United Kingdom

Oxford University Press is a department of the University of Oxford.
It furthers the University's objective of excellence in research, scholarship,
and education by publishing worldwide. Oxford is a registered trade mark of
Oxford University Press in the UK and in certain other countries

© Oxford University Press 2014

The moral rights of the author have been asserted

First Edition published in 2014

Impression: 1

All rights reserved. No part of this publication may be reproduced, stored in
a retrieval system, or transmitted, in any form or by any means, without the
prior permission in writing of Oxford University Press, or as expressly permitted
by law, by licence or under terms agreed with the appropriate reprographics
rights organization. Enquiries concerning reproduction outside the scope of the
above should be sent to the Rights Department, Oxford University Press, at the
address above

You must not circulate this work in any other form
and you must impose this same condition on any acquirer

Published in the United States of America by Oxford University Press
198 Madison Avenue, New York, NY 10016, United States of America

British Library Cataloguing in Publication Data
Data available

Library of Congress Control Number: 2013957077

ISBN 978–0–19–870487–4

Printed and bound in Great Britain by
CPI Group (UK) Ltd, Croydon, CR0 4YY

Oxford University press makes no representation, express or implied, that the
drug dosages in this book are correct. Readers must therefore always check
the product information and clinical procedures with the most up-to-date
published product information and data sheets provided by the manufacturers
and the most recent codes of conduct and safety regulations. The authors and
the publishers do not accept responsibility or legal liability for any errors in the
text or for the misuse or misapplication of material in this work. Except where
otherwise stated, drug dosages and recommendations are for the non-pregnant
adult who is not breast-feeding.

Links to third party websites are provided by Oxford in good faith and
for information only. Oxford disclaims any responsibility for the materials
contained in any third party website referenced in this work.

Acknowledgements

I would like to thank Dr Rebecca Ford for reading the manuscript and for her useful suggestions. Many thanks to Professor Michael Gleeson and Dr Stefan Brew for taking care of my physical health, and to Dr Antony Garelick for helping me develop a framework of understanding. These doctors saved me, and this book evolved as I recovered. Thanks to Ace for saving me from myself, and to my mother for her endless belief, love, and support. This book was only possible after time spent with colleagues discussing and considering these issues, in particular, Dr Alex Thomson. Thanks also to everyone at OUP, especially Chris Reid and Geraldine Jeffers for their enthusiasm, belief, and help in developing this project. This book is dedicated to my godchildren, Noah and Ako Kent.

Please contact me *@duncanharding* with any comments, tips, or suggestions. Use *#DTO* and contribute to our OSCE discussion.

Detailed contents

CHAPTER 1

Setting the scene

CONTENTS

A strategic approach

An objective structured clinical examination (OSCE) forms the practical component of most professional clinical examinations, and is generally considered to be the fairest standardized assessment of clinical skills and competencies.[1-4] I decided to write this book because there are common psychological hurdles to all OSCEs, and I think that, as a psychiatrist, I am well placed to suggest some psychological strategies for overcoming these.

I believe that it is possible to develop a generic way of approaching the different OSCE stations in every specialty that will increase confidence and improve the chance of success in *any* scenario. This may seem bold and ambitious, but actually is quite simple—it is simply a matter of deconstructing the scenarios into their component parts, and developing a personal skills toolkit that complements the competencies being tested. I will suggest ways of doing this.

This book is also intended to try to help those candidates who have already failed their OSCE examination, and are perhaps looking for a new approach for their subsequent attempt. Since the average OSCE pass rate of some of the Royal Colleges is in the region of 40–50%, this unfortunately is not an insignificant number.[5] The psychological component of failure and the baggage it produces should not be underestimated. This book directly addresses the unhelpful cognitions and beliefs that repeat candidates will have inevitably gained after failing, and helps them to understand and reframe that psychological baggage into something more positive.

Mechanics and organization

One size can never fit all, and there are subtleties and complexities to the different professions and specialties that make it impossible to generalize between them. However, there are core skills and anxieties common to all OSCEs, and these are often glossed over or neglected in other OSCE books. I will highlight these, and, in a way, this book is an extension of the first few pages in most undergraduate and postgraduate OSCE books that provide generic non-technical tips and strategies.

Some OSCEs use real patients, some use actors, and you may sometimes find yourself interacting with an inanimate object such as a mannequin. In a sense, all of these examples are simulated patients, since even the real patients will have probably taken part in many OSCEs and are essentially professionals in this role. The OSCE is a simulation of real life, and no matter who or what takes on the role of the simulated patient, they should be treated in exactly the same way—with upmost respect, compassion, and consideration. I tend to refer to the simulated patient as the *patient/actor*. This is for the purpose of reinforcing the importance of treating a simulated patient as *real*, whilst recognizing the fact that they are indeed *acting*. This conflict is also reflected in your own role in this artificial, time-limited OSCE simulation—you must be real, whilst recognizing the fact that you are acting. Recognizing and accepting this conflict is an important hurdle to overcome in this process.

Taking the OSCE seriously, and treating the simulated encounter as a real-life patient interaction, is crucial. In this way, you are entering into the spirit of the simulation, and you are playing your role within the scenario. The examiners are expecting you to take this encounter very seriously, and you must not disappoint them. However, the fact remains that we are pretending, and we need to recognize this and incorporate it into our mental preparation for the road ahead. I will address these issues later in this book.

You will also notice that I tend to use the word *scenario* rather than *station*. This is to reinforce the fact than an OSCE is a simulation of real life, and that even the most straightforward and practical of OSCE stations is actually simulating a real-life scenario. I will use anecdotes and examples throughout (see Box 1.1).

BOX 1.1 ANECDOTES AND EXAMPLES

I will use anecdotes and practical examples from the OSCE to illustrate key points and principles. These will be from personal experience and discussion with colleagues in my own and other specialties. As health practitioners, we are familiar by now with the ease by which factual information can be memorized when it is cognitively linked to a real clinical scenario— if you can attach an illness to a face, you will remember it. I hope that the anecdotes scattered throughout the text will help to explain the concepts discussed here and also act as trigger points for your memory and recall.

Process and content skills

Aside from the specific *content* skills required to navigate an OSCE scenario successfully, there are also some other more generic skills that are examined. These are *process* skills, and examples include professionalism, communication, listening, and empathy. We will spend some time considering process skills, and I will focus on your formation of a connection with the patient/actor. These non-technical skills are important because sometimes it is the processes that underlie and carry our OSCE performance that can let us down (particularly in those candidates on the borderline of success). Your content skills are obviously crucial for OSCE success, and for those you will need to look elsewhere. (They are specialty specific, and are the focus of most other OSCE books and online resources.) Whilst you will not find specific content skills here, we will consider ways, later in this book, that you can repackage your content skills into a more modular, transferrable form.

Being suspicious of the familiar

On the surface, an OSCE station may look identical to one that has appeared in previous sittings of the examination, and could seem to be familiar and straightforward. However, be suspicious of every single scenario, and don't be fooled into feeling comfortable or familiar with any. This time, there may be a new sinister problem lying below the surface—always scratch down to look for it; always probe deeper and screen wider to make sure you don't miss something serious. This is analogous to every single patient interaction you will ever have. We simply can't miss something sinister and serious in real life, and must always be vigilant and careful in even the most familiar of well-trodden clinical interactions.

So whilst I agree that using other OSCE material to prepare for and rehearse the scenarios that have already come up in the examination can be helpful, don't feel too secure with that, and please realize that every scenario is brand new to you and needs to be viewed with fresh eyes. Indeed, even if an OSCE scenario is identical to one that has appeared in the examination previously, it will have a different patient/actor and a different examiner. You will be examined by the way you interact in *this* situation, with *this* particular patient/actor. So even if you know all the required information, you still need to bounce your empathy and technique off whatever the patient/actor is giving you to work with. You need to be very sensitive to this particular patient/actor's anxieties and needs, and address them appropriately.

Generic skills and strategies

I believe that a person should walk into each OSCE scenario with no detailed plans, lists, or objectives, and that scenarios should be tackled with a clear head, fresh eyes, and open ears. Don't be burdened by knowing exactly what you will ask in a scenario. Use perhaps the most important skill in any OSCE to guide your investigation—*listening to the patient/actor*.

Enter your OSCE with a skills toolkit in your metaphorical back pocket, from which you can extract any tool you wish if you need it. Over-learning a scenario is like walking into the examination with the appropriate tools already in your hands, making it so much harder to fumble around and find the right tool if the scenario throws you a curve-ball. Approach each scenario with your hands empty and unburdened, and when you need a tool, dip into your back pocket and deftly extract the tool you need. This book will help you to build your own skills toolkit to carry with you in your examination.

We will also develop a generic strategy that will allow you to enter *any* OSCE station and find a way to move forwards. I suggest that you should enter a scenario with no more than five bullet points in your head. If the plan is any more robust and formulated than that, then you won't allow yourself the cognitive space to manoeuvre and adapt within the short time available to find the key to the scenario—and *finding the key* is the objective. You know once you've found the key and unlocked the scenario. You might not remember to say everything, but if you find the key and get to the bottom of a scenario, then you will probably be successful.

A time to reframe

- *Position one:* The OSCE is the gateway to the rest of your career, and is an opportunity for you to demonstrate your clinical skills to a senior peer group. It is also a fantastic opportunity for you to improve and refine those skills, both within your exam preparation study groups (when you will be demonstrating your skills to friends and colleagues for perhaps the first time) and also during the examination itself. If you fail the examination, you are often provided with feedback from each examiner. So even this is *formative* feedback, informing and improving your future performance.
- *Position two:* Some candidates reading this book have already failed their OSCE, and perhaps have experienced their examiners' feedback firsthand. I realize that this feedback might just

have made you feel bemused, confused, disheartened, and may even have left you feeling that the whole process is very unfair. I understand that you may think the OSCE is not a good test of your ability as a safe, successful health practitioner.

Therein lies the essence of the kind of psychological baggage and hurdles inherent in this process. If you approach the OSCE as in position one, you will probably perform better than if you take the stance in position two. This is because you will take the process more seriously, will be more motivated, and will perform very competitively against the more demoralized candidates who feel that it is all a waste of time. So whilst both positions may be valid to a certain extent, we should try tactically to reframe our approach and step back into the mind-set of the first position, rather than adopting the stance of the second. We will try to do that.

Framework of understanding

This book hopes to provide you with a framework of understanding. Normally when we experience life, we do not make efforts to separate thoughts from feelings, to dissect our beliefs from our underlying cognitions. However, there are times in life when it is useful to do so, and I suggest that the OSCE is one of those times. Many common illnesses, such as depression and anxiety, benefit from a more psychological approach to their treatment in the first instance. The basic principle of this treatment is to develop insight and understanding into our specific thoughts, feelings, and beliefs, and how these interact with each other. It is often useful, in itself, to examine our own psychological states more critically. When we become the investigators of ourselves, we are more able to take a step back and objectively dissect out the thoughts, feelings, and underlying beliefs that may be causing us difficulty. I will suggest ways of doing this.

Defining thoughts and cognitions

We will consider our thoughts. These are a product of mental activity resulting in an idea, opinion, or mental picture. Our thoughts may be singular or part of a thought process, and are usually linked to our feelings and beliefs. Our emotional state and underlying beliefs can dictate, create, modify, and distort our thoughts. In this book, I will suggest ways of accessing our blend of thoughts, beliefs, and emotions, in an attempt to extract our actual distinct thoughts. Sometimes our thoughts can be less than conscious and sometimes can be clouded by strong emotion. We will work together, however, to make our thoughts more conscious, distinct, and identifiable.

In this book, we will also consider our cognitions, often in the context of our *underlying* cognitions. When I ask colleagues the difference between thoughts and cognitions, they often reply with the view that these are essentially the same thing—hence this discussion. When we discuss cognition, we are considering a mental process, often less than conscious, underlying our conscious thoughts and feelings. Cognition is more than just a thought process: it is a process of understanding and acquiring knowledge, through thoughts and perceptions, feelings and intuition, and is often dictated and moulded by our core beliefs. Cognition describes an array of mental processes including attention, learning, problem solving, decision making, and memory. Cognition is the way that we understand and process the world around us.

When I describe underlying cognitions, I am considering the underlying, less than conscious mental processes that act to enable our understanding of the world, and these are often employing certain aspects of our beliefs and psychic development that are not overtly conscious and identifiable to us. We may, for example, harbour the belief that we are a 'failure'. In this case, our understanding of the world around us, our mental processing of perceptual cues, may be distorted by the core belief that we are a failure. If we believe, in our core, that we are a failure, then being criticized by an examiner may have a much deeper negative impact than if we truly believe that we are a 'success'.

It is too complex to try to dissect out and fully understand our underlying cognitions, and when I describe them, I am using a blanket term to describe all of the complex, less than conscious mental processes that occur when we make sense of the world around us. We can't change easily the way we process the world, but sometimes we may harbour an unhelpful belief that could tend to distort that processing. With the OSCE, especially once we have failed, we can develop unhelpful beliefs that may impinge on our cognitions—that is to say, impinge on our processing and understanding of the world. In this book, we will work together to access some of these underlying cognitions and beliefs, in order to try to understand why things might be going wrong and to consider how we might fix them.

The road ahead

So we will start our journey by updating our computer operating system, and we will attempt to identify and clean up any threats or viruses. We will be doing some structural work and strengthening our joists, beams, and foundations before we improve the decoration. We are looking under the bonnet of the car and retuning the engine before we fill up with petrol and try to drive faster than before. We will be constructing metal scaffolding that is solid and robust, onto which we can start to attach our process and content skills. With our new operating system, v2.0, we can face the OSCE with fresh eyes, unburdened by failures of the past, with confidence and self-belief. This is our objective.

In the first part of this book, we will consider the OSCE from a psychological perspective, looking at important issues such as psychological baggage, anxiety, and moving on after failure. In the next part of the book, we will look at more pragmatic issues relevant to your OSCE, such as OSCE construction, forming a connection with the patient, and study groups. Finally, we will explore how you can develop a skills toolkit and generic strategy for your OSCE. This is our road ahead, and our destination is success.

References

1. Harden, R. M. and Gleeson, F. A. (1979). Assessment of clinical competence using an Objective Structured Clinical Examination (OSCE). *Medical Education.* **13**: 41–54.
2. Sloan, D. A., Donnelly, M. B., Schwartz, R. W., and Strodel, W. E. (1995). The Objective Structured Clinical Examination. The new gold standard for evaluating postgraduate and clinical performance. *Annals of Surgery.* **222**: 735–42.
3. Davis, M. H. (2003). OSCE: the Dundee experience. *Medical Teacher.* **25**: 255–61.
4. Newble, D. (2004). Techniques for measuring clinical competence: objective structured clinical examinations. *Medical Education.* **38**: 199–203.
5. See the examination results reports from all of the different Royal Colleges, easily found on the internet. For example:
   a. MRCPsych Examinations Cumulative Results 2008-2010, *The Royal College of Psychiatrists.* (http://www.rcpsych.ac.uk/pdf/MRCPsych%20Cumulative%20Results%20Report%20-%20August%202011.pdf)
   b. Public Report on the Part 2 FRCOphth Examination February/April 2009, *The Royal College of Ophthalmologists.* (http://www.rcophth.ac.uk/core/core_picker/download.asp?id=599)
   c. Pass Rates for the MRCP(UK) Examination, *The Royal College of Physicians.* (http://www.mrcpuk.org/Results/Pages/ExamPassRates.aspx)
   d. Results, Allocations and Statistics, *The Royal College of Anaesthetists.* (http://www.rcoa.ac.uk/node/296)

CHAPTER 2

Carrying baggage

CONTENTS

Travel light

We all carry some psychological baggage with us into any situation, and the OSCE is no different. It is inevitable that we need to bring some carry-on baggage. However, rather than struggling to cram a big bag into an overhead locker, we should try to travel light and just bring a drink and maybe a magazine. This chapter will consider some of the different types of baggage that we carry with us into our OSCE, and suggests a way that you might consider and reframe your own baggage.

The good practitioner

A candidate who walks into their OSCE laden with heavy psychological baggage is at a disadvantage to a candidate who has none. This is because an OSCE is not just about delivering information or completing a task: it's actually a demonstration, to your senior colleagues, of your ability to function as a *good practitioner* (and being a good practitioner is much more than simply delivering information or finishing a task). A good practitioner makes a patient or relative feel safe and at ease. A good practitioner cares, communicates clearly, and is always understood. A good practitioner will look at the big picture and think holistically, whilst also investigating in depth. Patients are often vulnerable and misunderstood; so a good practitioner must protect them and understand them.

When you are examined in your OSCE, the examiner will often get a feel for whether or not you are a good practitioner, and this will depend critically on the way you conduct yourself and interact. If you are uncaring and don't listen to the patient, then you are a bad practitioner, no matter how much knowledge and information you can elicit or deliver, and a bad practitioner will not pass the OSCE. The gateway to career progression is guarded by the OSCE process, and bad practitioners need to be weeded out. Only good practitioners should be allowed to pass through.

Think of your driving test. The driving test examiner gets a feel for whether you are a good or bad driver. Passing through the gateway that he guards allows you to drive alone for the rest of your life, so only good drivers should be allowed to pass through. Whether you are a good or bad driver becomes apparent to the examiner by how safe they feel whilst you drive. If they feel unsafe, they will find a reason to fail you, even if your technique is very good. If they feel safe, they will be more forgiving of the small errors in your performance. Driving is a serious and potentially dangerous business (much like being a health practitioner), and the driving test examiner takes his gatekeeping role very seriously. Whether or not he perceives you to be a good and safe driver is dictated by the quality of your interaction with him, and, whilst he does use a standardized checklist to measure and report the quality of your driving, he will be guided actually by his gut feeling of whether or not you are safe. Such a gut feeling may be swayed by aspects of your performance in the test not easily measured and reported on a form. So, for example, if you appear reckless and arrogant, uncaring and overconfident, he may suspect that if you passed, you would be likely to cause serious harm whilst driving in your several tonnes' chunk of metal on a public road. Therefore, he may be extra critical and find a reason to back up his instinct with his standardized checklist appraisal. This isn't unfair; this is essential. If this didn't happen, and a person could pass the checklist and be successful even when the examiner felt unsafe, then we should all be very concerned to drive on the roads.

So how does carrying heavy baggage make you a bad practitioner? Well, in itself, it doesn't. However, it makes it so much harder for you to be a good practitioner in such an artificial, time-constrained setting, with noise in the background and bells ringing every few minutes. To be a good practitioner under OSCE conditions takes a particular state of mind, and carrying unnecessary psychological baggage makes it harder for us to achieve that state of mind.

Seeds of dissent

I was recently facilitating an OSCE study workshop, and a trainee joined our group. He started ranting on about how ridiculous it was that we give lots of money to the Royal College, only for them to stage the examination in a big, noisy hall with separate partitions, when surely they could afford to use real consultation rooms. He hadn't yet done his OSCE but was already carrying baggage; he was angry with the College and dismissive of the venue. I told him that he had to jettison those negative thoughts, and that his attitude wasn't good for the study group. He argued, but I pointed out that, unfortunately, the venue is only the tip of the iceberg of what one could get angry about with this process; there is much more valid stuff to be annoyed about. However, if you go into the examination annoyed about *any-thing*, you put yourself at a disadvantage before you even start. Why go into the OSCE burdened with negative thoughts and beliefs that put you at a disadvantage to others? Surely, if nothing else, the exam is too expensive for that? This particular person passed his OSCE first time with no problems, whereas several other people from the study group on that day failed. They didn't fail because of what he had said, but it annoyed me that he had infected our study group with his negative attitude, when he himself had no problems passing. Other candidates don't find it quite as easy to walk into their OSCE and pass with no problems. For them, things like a positive mental attitude and approach to the examination experience may be more important, because these things can improve performance.

So, as I will reiterate later, do not ever allow seeds of dissent into your study space, either from yourself or from others. This space needs to be a positive place, to allow good constructive study and preparation for this difficult examination.

Core internal state

To be successful in your OSCE, you need to walk into that examination venue with the right attitude, and this has to be something you believe down to your core, it can't be just an act. The scenarios are challenging, and while you are thinking and working with the patient/actor to complete the task at hand, the examiner will be watching closely. Your core internal state will shine out like a beacon—you can't hide it or disguise it. An area of concern for some of the Royal Colleges is *flippancy*, and if you walk into your OSCE thinking it is a waste of time, artificial, unfair, and stupid (and in the wrong venue), you can see easily how your core internal state of being flippant and unable to take the whole thing seriously will shine through. This may not be the case for every task, but it will certainly be true for the more challenging tasks. You can't hide your inner core in challenging tasks, and if you are expending energy trying to hide your contempt for the process, then you are diverting energy away from the challenging task at hand.

Being real

To be successful, you need to treat the interaction with the patient/actor as though it is a real patient interaction, and act as you would if you were alone in an Accident and Emergency Department on a Saturday night. You need to immerse yourself in this experience and take it very seriously. It is very hard to do that if you don't agree with it or think it's worthless. So you must break down your negative thoughts about your OSCE and reframe them into something more positive. I will suggest a way of doing this later.

The OSCE is a simulation of real life, and every OSCE strives to be as realistic as possible. You must play your role in this, and treat the experience as just another real-life clinical encounter. If this is difficult for you to do, you need to separate out your thoughts behind this and try to reframe them into something more helpful. Why can't you take this experience seriously? In fact, this encounter is a very significant clinical experience; one that will mould the rest of your career. Just because the 'patient' isn't 'real' doesn't matter. In some OSCEs, actual patients are used. However, since these patients have usually volunteered to assist in many previous OSCEs and are OSCE savvy, are they any more real than actors? At the end of the day, you are speaking to a person, and that is a real interaction.

The closer the OSCE can simulate a real clinical experience, the more powerful and useful that OSCE is as an assessment tool. However, you as a candidate have a role to play in that simulation of reality, and you must take the encounter and experience seriously. Examiner, patient/actor, and candidate all know this is just a simulation, but for this experience to have any value it needs to be taken very seriously. If you were an airline pilot in training, being examined in a flight simulator, you would have to take that simulation very seriously. If you didn't—and didn't immerse yourself in the experience by instilling it with as much reality as possible—then you would fail. It is the same for us. We are essentially being examined in a simulator, and if the examiner finds us competent, we will have patients' lives in our hands. The OSCE is the gateway to the rest of your training and career. It is very serious, and you need to take it seriously.

Reframing negative psychological baggage

So the objective for you now, before you even prepare for your OSCE, is to consider any negative thoughts you may have about it, reframe them into something more positive, and thereby put yourself in the strongest possible position for success. The reality is that no OSCE is perfect, but what in life is perfect? You need to deconstruct your negative baggage, and reframe it in your mind in a way that is more positive and healthy (see Exercise 2.1).

Over-rehearsal

Another type of baggage is over-rehearsal. Previous OSCE stations are available online and in books, and after you've completed the examination once, you will probably be familiar with the majority of possible scenarios. If you've already attempted the examination a couple of times, you will start to know

EXERCISE 2.1 REFRAMING BAGGAGE

Buy a notebook and dedicate it to excess and unwanted baggage (see Figure 2.1). At the top of each page, write a sentence that breaks the baggage down to its core. For example, the thoughts of the trainee I mentioned earlier might break down into: 'The venue is wrong; the College is ripping us off.'

Divide the page into three columns, and in the first column write your evidence for this. For example: 'The venue is too big and noisy, the setting isn't standardized, and the cubicles are artificial. The amount of money that this costs should surely be able to pay for a proper venue? If the exam is so important, then why aren't we examined in a more controlled and quiet setting?'

Try to capture the essence of the baggage in the title of the page and the content of the first column. If you wanted to explain to a friend why this particular aspect is so unfair, then the title and first column should be enough for them to read and really understand where you are coming from. It is important that you fully express your anger and frustration.

In the middle column, write down the harsh reality of the situation, as you understand it, whether it is fair or not. For example, you could write something like: 'The venue they use is the only venue big enough to stage the OSCE, with all the necessary stations and circuits, with holding areas, and with the facility to put through the necessary volume of candidates in a short time. The exam needs to be all finished in a short time period (days), to keep it as similar and standardized as possible for all candidates.'

This middle column won't make you feel any better, and may raise more questions. For example, why not hold the exam in a smaller venue, over more days? The middle column must be the rational explanation for the baggage in the title. If you don't know the rational reason, perhaps ask a colleague or supervisor. Or even email the College.

The last column is the most important, and shouldn't be completed straightaway; it needs to be thought about. You need to reframe the negative thoughts in a positive way that makes sense to you, and that you really believe in and identify with. It is the third column that will allow you to check in this baggage into the hold, instead of carrying it with you onto the flight. An example of the third column might be: 'The venue is a lot like a busy and noisy Accident and Emergency Department on a Saturday night, when you are assessing a patient in a flimsy curtained cubicle, and when your ability to spot red flags and sinister underlying problems and symptoms is ever more important. The OSCE venue simulates these conditions very well'. With the third column, you will reframe the negative thoughts into something more useful and positive.

the scenarios by heart. This is one of the worst and most dangerous types of baggage to carry into the examination. Whilst the OSCE scenarios are often repeated, there will usually be subtle but important differences in subsequent versions. The problem with already knowing what is needed for a particular scenario is that you are more likely to miss something new and subtle (see example in Box 2.1).

To be successful, the candidate must listen to every word and follow every lead. This is the key to success in any OSCE—*listening*. The candidate who knows a scenario too well will be thinking of what to say next and where they are going with the assessment. This is important, but it is much more important to be guided by the patient and listen very carefully to every single word.

I would suggest that if you ever walk into an OSCE station and think that you already know the answer, something is wrong. You should never know the answer to an OSCE scenario from the

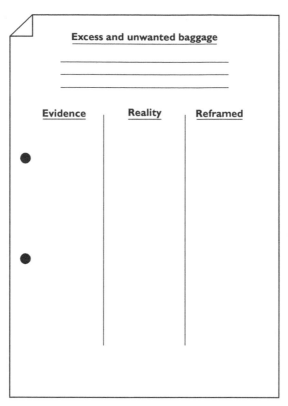

Figure 2.1 Excess and unwanted baggage
Break down and reframe unhelpful psychological baggage. See Appendix, Figure A.1.

BOX 2.1 TREAD CAREFULLY

For example, a regularly repeated psychiatry OSCE scenario involves a pregnant, breast-feeding mother who is depressed. It appears on the surface that this scenario is testing your knowledge of antidepressant medication. However, this scenario can play out in several different ways. Sometimes it has been straightforward, and a successful candidate should decide appropriate medication and discuss this with the husband. Sometimes, the mother has actually been psychotic, believing that her baby is a demon who she must kill. The psychosis is very subtle and difficult to identify, but once identified, the successful candidate should go on to tell the husband that his wife must be admitted under the Mental Health Act. Consequently, the husband gets furious and starts shouting (thereby testing the candidate's ability to deal with an angry relative). On other occasions, the depressed mother has actually been delusional, believing her baby to be terminally ill, and planning to 'save' it (by killing it). In this last example, if the candidate was aware of the possibility of an underlying psychosis and the risk of harm to the baby, they might miss the delusion and her plans to save it. Indeed, the mother admits no plans to harm her baby; she just wants to save her ill baby (by killing it). In each of these versions of the scenario, the initial instructions to the candidate are almost identical. Over-rehearsing the scenario a particular way is not only pointless, it decreases the chance of being able to solve the actual scenario on the day.

start, and if you feel confident, relieved, and comfortable with a well-trodden scenario, then you should tread even more carefully. The appropriate starting point is nearer to fear and confusion, rather than fearlessness and clarity. Perhaps an exaggeration, but please tread carefully.

Physical examinations

Some OSCE scenarios, such as physical examinations, do require lots of rehearsal and refinement of technique. The examination should appear second nature and seamless, and that level of proficiency can only be achieved through repeated practice. However, the candidate should still observe and listen very carefully, and must not just slip comfortably into a well-rehearsed technique (see Box 2.2).

BOX 2.2 FAMILIAR PHYSICAL EXAMINATIONS

For example, a candidate in the MRCP OSCE (PACES) may have rehearsed the 'eye examination' to perfection, and, when faced with proptosis, may run elegantly through the eye movements and examination of the fundus. However, they may miss a subtle clue in the patient's demeanour, and, therefore, may not think laterally enough to question them about thyroid activity status. So, whilst rehearsal is critical in physical examinations and the more practical of OSCE stations, still the candidate must avoid the pitfalls of a too well-furrowed pathway. They should always take an objective step backwards and think beyond the obvious task at hand.

Presenting findings

There may also be a tendency for the over-rehearsed to only present findings to the examiner that they think the examiner wants to hear. Beware of ignoring a clinical finding or line of questioning because it seems to go against what you were expecting to find in a particular scenario. You are unlikely to lose marks for commenting on additional findings, so long as they are not wrong (see Box 2.3).

BOX 2.3 ADDITIONAL FINDINGS

A colleague of mine gave me an example of this, when she was asked, in her medical short cases, to observe a patient's face and comment on her findings. The patient had the telangiectasia of Osler–Weber–Rendu syndrome, but also had a large esotropia. Even though this was obvious, none of her competitors had commented on it previously during that day. By mentioning that she would like to exclude a sixth nerve palsy as the cause of the convergent squint, my colleague almost certainly put the examiner in a favourable mood with her for the rest of the scenario.

Please try to think about the baggage you carry with you, even if that baggage makes you feel more confident about the OSCE (for example, over-rehearsal). Confidence can be your ally, but also your downfall if you miss something subtle. Never be comfortable with a scenario—always listen, look, and think about what you actually see in front of you. Above all, enter your OSCE with as clean a slate as possible, and don't allow your negative thoughts, beliefs, and preconceptions to disadvantage you against other less psychologically burdened candidates.

Further reading

1. Grosz, S. (2013). *The Examined Life: How We Lose and Find Ourselves*. Chatto and Windus, London. (Excellent book: useful when reflecting on the importance of underlying psychological issues in day-to-day life, and a good starting point to reflect on your own psychological baggage.)

CHAPTER 3

Moving on after failure

CONTENTS

Moving on

One of my motivations for writing this book was to try to consider the candidate who has perhaps already failed their OSCE, and to think of cognitive strategies that might be helpful for them. As the pass rate for the OSCE in some Royal Colleges is in the order of 40–50%, the numbers failing can be substantial.[1] The OSCE can be a difficult examination to pass, and it can become harder to pass with each successive attempt (for example, see[1a]). The reasons it can become harder are undoubtedly complex and multi-factorial, but the psychological components of this phenomenon are important to consider. We will look at the psychological aspects of OSCE failure in this chapter, and consider ways to move beyond these.

Grieving your loss

It is simply impossible for me to reframe your failure in the OSCE in any way that is wholly positive, and I wouldn't dare to try. I know that failure in this process is devastating and very expensive, and, like anything in life, you will need a period in which to grieve your loss. It worries me when a candidate who has failed does not seem unduly bothered by this, because failing this examination is upsetting and sometimes emotionally devastating. After all, we are all working or training as practitioners, assessing patients and managing risk, day in and day out. We have all been successful in gaining our training positions, and we have all passed the written papers. A health practitioner is a highly selected professional who has probably passed most of the examinations they have ever attempted. The selection process for training is extremely competitive, and we all have a good track record and many strings to our bows. So, failing the OSCE is often quite a shock.

Allow yourself time to grieve, and share this grief with friends, colleagues, and family. Don't be ashamed of your grief—allow it to wash through you. Allow yourself to progress through the normal stages of grief: denial; anger; bargaining; depression; and, finally, acceptance. Be aware that this is normal, and be open about it with others. Denying your grief will allow the possibility of your grieving process becoming abnormal or blocked at a particular stage. With the OSCE, you may find yourself denying your initial poor performance, and then becoming angry when you eventually get the results. You may get stuck in the anger stage, particularly if that anger is reinforced by a developing belief that the OSCE is flawed and worthless as an assessment tool. Don't let this happen. Let your mind progress through the stages of grief, and facilitate this process by speaking about it to others. If you allow yourself to be weak, you will regain your strength. Denial of your weakness will maintain it.

Being objective

Failure is very difficult to deal with, and there are two components to this that need to be carefully segregated in your mind—the *objective facts* and the *feelings*. It is probably useful to go over the details of the examination and try to work out what went wrong. This could be aided by examiner feedback if your institution provides that. However, try to be objective about the details, and view them as you would if you were helping a colleague. Don't let your emotions cloud your objectivity. We will think about your feelings separately, but, for now, we will consider the facts objectively.

It could be useful to think about the details of your failure with a colleague, perhaps in your study group, or perhaps with a colleague in the same situation. If you do this, try to remain dispassionate and objective. Treat the experience in the same way you would treat a challenging real-life clinical experience, and go over the details in the way you would speak about those specific real-life circumstances. Try not to let any emotional content infect your analysis of the facts, because this can cloud your objectivity.

You need to analyse what went wrong, but don't be burdened by this analysis. Don't let it sit on your shoulders. By analysing it and discussing it, you can get it out of your system and kick it into touch. A difficult clinical scenario can haunt you if you keep it locked inside, so it will be useful to talk through the details. If you manage to dissect out particular details that cause you difficulty—for example, perhaps you realize that you have a tendency to jump to diagnostic conclusions too early and, thereby, miss things because you are too focussed and single-minded—you can then work on these in your study group. It would be useful if the group were aware of such difficulties.

Your realizations regarding your analysis of the facts may be weighed down and distorted by an underlying belief or preconception—for example: 'this exam is an unfair assessment of my skills'. If you have an underlying belief that the OSCE is unfair, then this casts an unhelpful shadow over *any* realizations you may have otherwise made. For example: jumping to diagnostic conclusions too early may be a real problem for you, but this could be masked by the over-shadowing belief that the OSCE is simply an unfair and inadequate assessment of your skills. With such a negative underlying belief, it is much harder to dissect out objectively the real problems that led to failure. Often, such an underlying negative belief is actually a psychological defence mechanism that protects our ego from the pain of failure.

The pass zone

You shouldn't focus on what went wrong in the individual scenarios, though the College feedback regarding this may be useful and illuminating. Your next OSCE will be totally different, and you need to improve your overall functioning in the examination to ensure that you are in the 40–50% of candidates that pass next time. Don't dwell on the one scenario that you failed, that you feel was marked unfairly, and that, on its' own, prevented you from passing the OSCE. This is unhelpful (even if true).

Think of your OSCE as a driving test. If you need to do the test again, at the very least, you will definitely be a better driver. If you failed your test by not looking in the mirror, you can make sure you look in the mirror next time—but you may forget to cancel your indicator next time.

So, you shouldn't focus on the minutiae of what went wrong last time. You need to take a step back and look at the bigger picture. Remember that you don't have to pass all of the stations, and, even within a particular scenario, you don't have to do absolutely everything that the examiner might be looking for. You do, however, need to demonstrate to the examiner, and the process as a whole, that you are a good and safe practitioner, and you need to make sure that you are far enough into the 'pass zone' so that small mistakes or omissions don't land you in the 'fail zone'.

Consider your feelings

As a psychiatrist, I am well used to considering my feelings in a professional context, but trainees in other specialties may not be as familiar with this. It is always useful to have a good understanding of your feelings. This can inform your understanding of a patient, and can protect you if you have a difficult and distressing clinical experience. At the very least, we are all human beings, and our feelings will inevitably leak into our clinical practice. To remain dispassionate and objective in our job as effective practitioners, we need to understand them.

Failure makes us feel terrible, and it is important to realize that feeling terrible is very normal in this situation. Failure in the OSCE, if we take the OSCE seriously, makes us feel as though we are unworthy of our professional careers—and yet we must go back to work on Monday and reclaim responsibility of patients' lives and well-being. Our defence to this is to not take the OSCE seriously after failure. The way we can go back to our day job confidently and unburdened with our failure is to think that the OSCE is: inadequate; a bad examination; an unreliable way of assessing clinical skills. I know I am good and safe: I must be because I care for patients every day. Therefore, the OSCE must be *flawed* in some way. There may be some truth to this view, but adopting this stance is a problem because the best way to pass an OSCE is to take it seriously, treating it as a real scenario that has value and worth. As I said in the last chapter, your core internal state will shine through in a difficult scenario, so you will help yourself if you believe in the OSCE as a good examination of clinical skills and approach it seriously. This clashes with our feelings of failure and our need to go back to our day job on Monday to look after patients.

Being aware of your feelings, and understanding the conflict between knowing that you are a safe practitioner whilst accepting that you failed the OSCE, is the first step towards resolution. There is no absolute resolution between these conflicting positions, but being aware of the conflict is, in itself, helpful. The important thing is to not let yourself fall into the trap of believing that the OSCE is worthless, because you will be competing against first-timers who are taking the process more seriously since they believe it has true value.

Trauma

Traumatic events can result in the formation of unhelpful underling beliefs, and, if left unchecked, these beliefs can cause further difficulties in life (see a personal example in Box 3.1).

Failing the OSCE is a traumatic event. Think about the beliefs that you may have formed regarding the OSCE. Perhaps, after failing, you believe that the timing of the stations is not a realistic measure of normal clinical practice? Perhaps you believe that your Royal College is prejudiced in some way, or just trying to generate money? After failing the OSCE, it is likely that you have formed a belief that allows you to continue practicing as a 'success', with your head held high. Indeed, this is necessary.

In my example of trauma, my belief that I was going to get mugged again was reinforced every time I travelled safely by bus. There may have been some truth to this belief, but I was exaggerating that

> **BOX 3.1 A PERSONAL TRAUMA**
>
> A few years ago, I was mugged whilst walking home from my local tube station. This really scared me, and made me reluctant to go outside. I started getting a bus from the tube instead of taking the usual ten-minute walk home. I had developed the belief that I would be mugged again. I had lived there for eight years and never been mugged before, but, after the trauma, I believed that it would happen again. By getting the bus home, I was reducing my anxiety, but reinforcing the belief that if I walked home I would be mugged again. This psychological process was pointed out to me by a work colleague, and so I decided to challenge this belief by walking home. I felt extremely anxious, especially when I got to the place where I had previously been mugged. However, as I walked on, and didn't get mugged, I felt a weight lift off my shoulders. I had challenged the belief that I would get mugged, and provided myself with powerful contrary evidence.

truth, and, by focussing on it, I was not allowing myself to deal with the real underlying trauma. By changing my behaviour and breaking that cognitive link—I didn't get the bus, and walked—I explicitly challenged the belief. By getting the bus, I wasn't allowing myself to challenge the belief.

You need to identify any underlying beliefs that may be fuelling your feelings and emotions, and challenge them explicitly. There may be some truth to your beliefs, but you should dissect them out and try to understand them. This is because the beliefs are probably exaggerated and unhelpful, and you may be reinforcing them by your actions and behaviours, thereby making the beliefs even more entrenched within your mind. Challenge them.

The OSCE is flawed?

If you have previously failed the OSCE, then you may have formed the belief that the examination is flawed in some way. This belief is important to you because it allows you to continue working as a safe and competent practitioner. It is a psychological defence, protecting your ego from the painful reality of your failure. However, the belief may sabotage any future attempt at the OSCE, because it will not allow you to take the examination as seriously. Even if there is some truth to this belief—and indeed, perhaps, the OSCE is flawed in some ways—we must recognize that, by focussing on this, we are putting ourselves at a selective disadvantage, and we are also not allowing ourselves to deal with the real underlying issues that are causing us pain after failing the OSCE.

If failure in the OSCE has led to the belief, for example, that the OSCE is flawed, then this belief is potentially reinforced with every positive and successful patient encounter. If you are a good practitioner, how can the OSCE assessment of your abilities *not* be flawed? Every time a patient thanks you for a job well done, this should, in fact, add water to your internal reservoir of positivity that would normally help you through your clinical examinations. However, if you are a 'failure' in the eyes of the OSCE, whilst being praised for being a 'success' in the eyes of a patient or colleague, then this water can bypass your reservoir of positivity and, instead, fill the pool of new evidence that proves the OSCE is indeed a flawed process. This new belief that you have formed allows you to comfortably exist in a state of 'failure' and 'success'. However, if you could take away this unhelpful belief, you would allow the water to flow in the right direction.

You must break the cognitive link between your success as a practitioner and your belief that the OSCE is flawed (or whatever your specific belief may be). These are separate concepts. The link between the two protects your ego and allows you to resolve the fact that you are a 'failure' at the same time as being a 'success'. Exercise 3.1 is an opportunity to challenge your beliefs.

EXERCISE 3.1 CHALLENGING YOUR BELIEFS

Draw two horizontal lines onto a piece of A4 paper, dividing it into three equal sections. Label the top section, 'I failed the OSCE'; the middle section, 'The OSCE is flawed' (or whatever your specific belief may be); and the bottom section, 'I am a good practitioner' (see Figure 3.1).

Recording

In the top section, you should start by writing down the thoughts that are associated with the fact that you have failed the OSCE—not your feelings, just the actual thoughts. Put these thoughts in the upper part of the top section (you will be writing your feelings in the lower part). Spread the words out as you write them into each section of the page, and draw a circle around each word. The thoughts associated with failure are often very difficult to filter out from the feelings because they are loaded with emotion. Examples might be: 'expensive', 'time-consuming', 'delayed training', 'my friend passed'. Try to distil out the objective thoughts that occur to you when you think of your failure. Draw a line under these. Underneath, write down your honest feelings associated with your failure in the OSCE. This will be much easier, but may be painful. Examples might be: 'disappointed', 'embarrassed', 'ashamed'. Draw connecting lines between the words that are linked in some way. For example, you may draw a line between the thought that 'my friend passed' and the feeling of 'embarrassment'. Make the cognitive links between the thoughts and the feelings. You now have a more structured understanding of your thoughts and feelings associated with your failure in the OSCE, and the cognitive links between these.

In the middle section of the page, consider your belief that the OSCE is flawed (or whatever specific belief you have formed), and at the top of this section write down the thoughts that come to mind. For example, these might be: 'rushed', 'artificial', 'unfair'. You are trying objectively to capture a description of your belief about the OSCE. Draw a line under this. Next, underneath this, write down the feelings that the OSCE invokes. Examples might be: 'frustration', 'anger', 'sadness'. Try to capture how the OSCE makes you feel. Then, draw lines between any of the words in the middle section that are linked. For example, you may feel that your thought that the OSCE is 'unfair' directly links to your feelings of 'sadness', whereas the word 'artificial' might link to 'frustration', 'anger', and 'sadness'. Try to link the thoughts with the feelings, and understand these links. In the middle section of the page you have broken down your belief about the OSCE into thoughts and feelings, and you have tried to understand the cognitive links between these. You now have a more robust understanding of your belief.

In the bottom section of the page, write down the thoughts that occur to you when you think of yourself as a good practitioner. These might be words that capture the evidence that allows you to think this. For example, you might write: 'safe', 'caring', 'conscientious'. Draw a line under these. Underneath, write down the feelings you get when you think of yourself as a good practitioner. Examples might be: 'happy', 'proud', 'satisfied,'. Draw lines between the words in the lower section of the page that are linked—you are making the explicit links between the thoughts and the feelings associated with you being a good practitioner. For example, you may draw a line between the words 'safe' and 'proud'. Think about the links, and think about your belief that you are a good practitioner. Think about all the patients who would agree with this, and try to think of particular patients who would agree with particular thoughts. For example, you might have had a recent encounter where you were particularly caring towards a patient, and, if asked, they might strongly agree with your view that you are caring. The bottom section of the page should capture the truth of you as a practitioner, and should be imbued with memories of actual clinical encounters. You have captured the belief of yourself as a good practitioner,

(continued)

and now have a more robust understanding of the thoughts and feelings that constitute this belief.

Reflecting

Look at the page, and look at the content of the top and bottom sections—they are not compatible. They clash. They don't make sense together. This is because your failure in the OSCE does not sit comfortably next to your success as a practitioner.

The middle section of the page (for example, your belief that the OSCE is flawed) allows the top and bottom sections of the page to coexist comfortably. However, you must try to disregard the middle section of the page, and you need to challenge your belief that the OSCE is flawed. It is not enough to write a 'pros and cons' list and challenge this belief with written facts. This won't work, because the belief is essential in allowing the coexistence of the opposing forces of failure and success.

The bottom section of the page (you being a good practitioner) fuels and reinforces your belief that, for example, the OSCE is flawed, and allows you to continue failing the OSCE while you continue to be a good practitioner. You must bypass this cognitive link; sever the links between being a good practitioner and your belief that the OSCE is flawed. Do this symbolically by drawing a thick line between the middle and bottom sections of the page.

We could, probably, draw links between the content of the bottom and middle sections of the page—but we will not do that. Rather, we will recognize that reinforcing the belief that the OSCE is flawed is profoundly unhelpful, given that we need to pass the OSCE in the future.

Instead, take a red pen, and look at the content of the top and bottom sections of the page. Draw lines that link the words in these two sections, bypassing the middle section. For example, the word 'safe' in the bottom section is evidence that you are a good practitioner, but it also makes you feel even more disappointed that you failed in the OSCE, so link the word 'safe' with 'disappointment'. Think about this cognitive link, and how the evidence and feelings from the bottom section of the page (that you are a good practitioner) make the feelings in the top section of the page (that you failed) stronger and more painful. Indeed, if you weren't a safe practitioner, perhaps you wouldn't feel quite as disappointed by your failure? Make strong cognitive links between the bottom and top sections of the page, and bypass the middle section (the belief that the OSCE is flawed) altogether. This belief is not only unhelpful, it is also too easy. It is the easy way out of trying to reconcile your failure with your success, and it is lazy and actually wrong. Make strong links between your abilities as a practitioner and your failure in the OSCE, and try to understand how your success actually fuels your feelings associated with failure. Our successful patient encounters will start to challenge the thoughts and feelings associated with failing the OSCE, instead of reinforcing the belief that the OSCE is flawed. You need to make those new links and reject your unhelpful beliefs about the OSCE. Use your positive encounters and experience to explicitly challenge and contradict the baggage created by failure, instead of allowing them to implicitly reinforce an unhelpful underlying internal and often insidious belief.

Finally, you can write a few words in the middle section that challenge your belief that the OSCE is flawed, but write these last, and draw a square around each word to distinguish them. This is the icing on the cake. The hard work has already been done, but a few words to challenge the belief will be helpful.

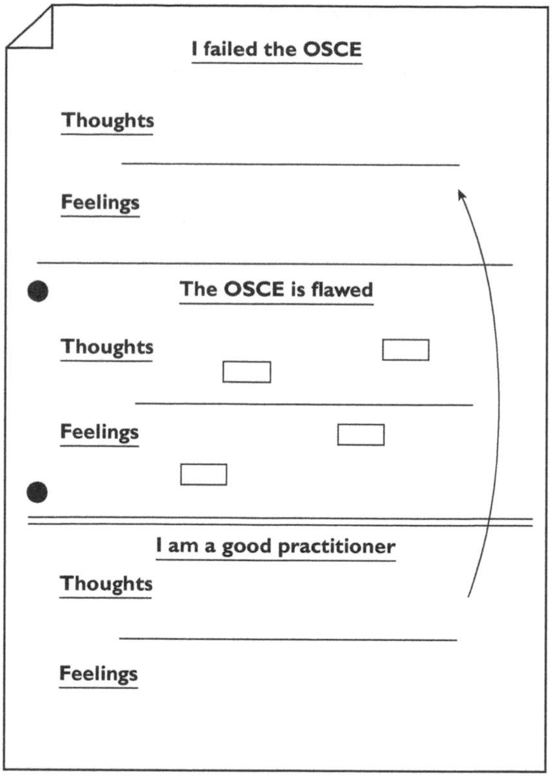

Figure 3.1 Challenging your beliefs

Explore and bypass those unhelpful beliefs that resolve the conflict of 'failure' and 'success'. See Appendix, Figure A.2.

Group support

It may be useful to try to think about the emotions surrounding your failure in a more objective way, and take a step back, assessing your feelings from the perspective of someone else. Openly discuss your feelings within your study group. If a member of the group volunteers how they are feeling, ask them why they feel this way. Consider why you might feel this way, and try to identify the thoughts that are driving your feelings. Challenge your feelings and emotions. Why do you feel inadequate? Don't gloss over this—actively dissect into your group's feelings and write down the evidence that backs them up, or the facts that challenge them. Try to identify and reframe the underlying beliefs that drive the thoughts and feelings. You are not inadequate. There is lots of evidence to back up the fact that you are not inadequate. Remove the shroud of secrecy, and consider this openly as a group.

The value of change

Spending energy on refining process skills (such as empathy), as I suggest later in this book, may feel like a waste of time when preparing for subsequent examination attempts, and your anxiety would perhaps be more abated by devoting time to perfecting the required content skills. However, knowing that you have changed your strategy and systems is, in itself, very helpful psychologically, as you are not just re-treading the same boards. You are not just trying to drive the same car faster. You are actually now driving a different but faster car. You are rebooting your system, wiping the slate clean, and losing some of the anxiety surrounding things that went wrong last time, because this time, things will be *different*.

You need to rethink your strategy and approach, and start from scratch. Forget the preparation you did before; this time you will be doing something totally different. That in itself will give you hope and strength, because if you just prepare in the same way, what will change from before? Changing your whole approach to your OSCE will allow you to tackle the process from a different perspective. You will still have the strengths acquired during your previous preparation and attempts, but you will also have this totally new angle and approach.

Also, don't forget, if you have failed your OSCE, then actually you have done the best and most brutal mock OSCE examination that you could ever do. If you have failed a few times, then you have done a few mock OSCEs. You have experienced the whole process, and are prepared in a way that will elude first-timers. You know exactly what to expect, and you will not be thrown or distracted by this unusual and unique process and experience.

References

1. See the examination results reports from all of the different Royal Colleges, easily found on the internet. For example:
   a. MRCPsych Examinations Cumulative Results 2008–2010, *The Royal College of Psychiatrists*. (http://www.rcpsych.ac.uk/pdf/MRCPsych%20Cumulative%20Results%20Report%20-%20 August%202011.pdf)
   b. Public Report on the Part 2 FRCOphth Examination February/April 2009, *The Royal College of Ophthalmologists*. (http://www.rcophth.ac.uk/core/core_picker/download.asp?id=599)
   c. Pass Rates for the MRCP(UK) Examination, *The Royal College of Physicians*. (http://www. mrcpuk.org/Results/Pages/ExamPassRates.aspx)
   d. Results, Allocations and Statistics, *The Royal College of Anaesthetists*. (http://www.rcoa.ac.uk/ node/296)

Reframing anxiety

CONTENTS

Anxiety

Anxiety affects us all, in many different situations in life. In the OSCE, it is useful to consider that the nature and purpose of anxiety is essentially positive: it increases our attention and focus towards a particular problem; it raises our arousal and psychomotor activity; it boosts adrenaline and, so, improves our performance. It allows us to engage with a difficulty in a heightened way, with the intention of us overcoming that hurdle and moving on in life. However, anxiety can very easily make us shift into a darker place. It can feel very unpleasant, and, what was an excited, heightened bodily state, can effortlessly turn into something more negative that feels bad and wrong.

The OSCE is an important hurdle for a health practitioner, and success means career progression. This has financial, social, and psychological implications, and passing the OSCE is extremely important for all of us. In our first attempt, we feel anxious. This anxiety will help us usually to perform better and improve our chance of success. For a few people, the anxiety will be overwhelming, even during the first ever attempt, and will become a hindrance to success. When a candidate has failed the OSCE once (for whatever reason), they will feel naturally more anxious in their subsequent attempts, with this anxiety much more likely to become overpowering and counter-productive. The importance of the OSCE is such that this increase in anxiety cannot but feel unpleasant—too much rests on the need for success.

The interesting thing about OSCE-related anxiety is that a candidate can reduce this, during preparation, by immersing themselves in the required content skills. This book will not relieve anxiety as effectively as a book filled with the actual information required to pass your particular OSCE, and I can understand candidates much preferring to use those kinds of books. However, the irony is that anxiety demonstrates itself to your examiners by your *process* skills, rather than the content skills. The way you interact and present yourself betrays your anxiety in a way that the content never can. So, whilst learning the content may make you feel better in the short term, it won't address, necessarily, the way that your anxiety is actually affecting your OSCE performance. You need to understand your anxiety, and then think about the way it affects your presentation, for example, by making your hands fidget or shake.

I suggest that anxiety is a useful and essential tool for OSCE success, and, in fact, the more times you fail, the more anxious you get, the better you are equipped for this examination. This may sound hollow and patronizing, but I believe it to be true. I just think that a little more thought needs to go into the anxiety surrounding the OSCE. It needs to be reframed in a way that removes the negative associated cognitions, leaving the anxiety performing its natural function—improving your performance.

A cognitive model

Earlier in this book, I described my own experience of being mugged to illustrate how a traumatic event can lead to an underlying belief (that I would be mugged again) that is then reinforced by subsequently modified behaviour (catching the bus home instead of walking). Every bus journey reinforced my underlying belief that I would be mugged again. This underlying belief made me feel more anxious and was a distorted, exaggerated, and unhelpful belief. In fact, I had lived there for eight years and never been mugged before. When I became aware of this (through a work colleague), I explicitly challenged this belief by forcing myself to walk home. I changed my behaviour. I felt more anxious in the short term, and, indeed, I had removed the behaviour (catching the bus) that was acting to significantly *reduce* my anxiety. However, as I passed the point in the street where I had been mugged, I felt a weight lift off my shoulders. I found contrary evidence to challenge the belief that I would be mugged—I walked home and I wasn't mugged. If I had continued using the bus, this belief would have grown and, possibly, become entrenched within me. I dissected it out though, and challenged it by changing my behaviour.

Let us again consider failure in the OSCE. Once you fail the OSCE (or, sometimes, before you even attempt it for the first time), you naturally develop a fear of failure. This is perfectly normal and to be expected. However, if we examine this fear a little more closely, we realize that there is an underlying belief driving the fear. This belief could be something like: 'I will fail again' or 'I am a failure'. There is usually no smoke without fire, and there is usually no fear without an underlying belief driving that fear. The strength of conviction of the underlying belief 'I will fail again' dictates how problematic the resulting anxiety will become. No matter how confident a candidate is, they will naturally fear failure after they have failed once already. Also, don't forget that this may be the first time a candidate has ever failed an examination. That is perhaps partly why a first-time candidate who believes they will pass has an advantage over a candidate who has already failed. The retaking candidate has started to form an underlying belief that they will fail again, and this cognitive state then has repercussions for their subjective experience of anxiety. It pushes the natural (and useful) anxiety into a darker place.

Anxiety experienced whilst also having an underlying belief that you will fail is distorted into evidence that reinforces the underlying belief. The candidate feels anxious, and this anxiety is evidence that things will go wrong again. Anxiety can give us a sense of dread, and anxiety combined with an underlying belief that you will fail increases the chance of experiencing dread. You can see how difficult it is to experience anxiety in a positive, performance-enhancing way when you believe, deep down, that you will fail again. Therefore, we must reframe our experience of anxiety and challenge our underlying belief that we will fail again. What is the evidence that we will fail again? Indeed, since we have already taken the examination at least once before, and we have practised and studied for another six months, surely our chances of failure have reduced? It is very important to address your underlying beliefs once you have failed, and to challenge them.

Anxiety is a positive psychological state that can help us in this examination. We must embrace anxiety, not reject it. We must understand that feeling anxious is normal, and should be incorporated into our performance and preparation. We know that, on the day, our anxiety will increase our arousal, make us think faster on our feet, and improve our chances of success. Embrace your anxiety (see Box 4.1).

BOX 4.1 **EMBRACING ANXIETY**

A colleague of mine, who is a singer, told me that having no anxiety results in a lacklustre performance, giving the impression that you don't care about the music. However, too much anxiety can make you lose your tuning and forget your words. So, a good singer needs just the right amount of anxiety for the perfect performance.

We must understand our underlying beliefs, and be aware that there are things that reinforce those beliefs, and things that can challenge them.

Challenging unhelpful beliefs

As I mentioned previously (see Chapter 3), once we have failed an OSCE, we are in the strange position of being a 'failure' alongside, simultaneously, being a 'success'. We usually resolve this contradiction by forming the belief (or opinion) that the OSCE is in some way a flawed examination, and that it does not allow you adequately to demonstrate (or measure) your success. We are a success because the day after the failed OSCE, we are back at work, seeing and treating patients. We are on-call, working on the front line. How would an establishment let us treat patients if we were a failure? Indeed, we know that we are a success because, despite whatever the OSCE examiner may think, our patients like us and feel happy with our service and their treatment.

We can use this to our advantage. If we can shed the unhelpful, ego-preserving belief that the OSCE is a flawed process (see Chapter 3), then we can divert any positive-affirming clinical encounters and experiences into our internal reservoir of confidence and strength. Moving on to our possible deeper, more painful, and unhelpful belief that 'I will fail in the OSCE'—the second you perform in real life as a successful health practitioner, this is powerful evidence that your underlying fear and negative belief is false. Allow the positive-affirming water to flow the right way, into your reservoir of positivity. Every on-call, every procedure, every patient interaction is all evidence that can be used to challenge your underlying belief that you are a failure and to show, instead, that you are clearly a success.

However, in order for this to have any cognitive weight, you should be aware of your underlying beliefs, and you must consciously challenge these beliefs with contrary evidence. If I hadn't explicitly considered my underlying belief that I would be mugged again, and actually thought about the reinforcement that was occurring by my travelling home on the bus, I would not have had such a powerful reaction to challenging that belief by walking home. If I was oblivious to the underlying cognitive theoretical construct, I may actually have added to the belief that I would be mugged again by walking home instead of catching the bus (because I felt more anxious). However, by consciously thinking about these issues, and then choosing to walk home (even though that made me feel a lot more anxious), I had a very powerful psychological reaction that helped to challenge my underlying belief that I would be mugged again.

Unhelpful underlying beliefs can interact with your thoughts and feelings in a complex way. Your underlying cognitions (the way you process the world) can be distorted by these complex interactions. There may be several different aspects of your underlying cognitions that are unhelpful, such as your thought processes (conscious and less than conscious) perhaps driven by your belief structures. It might be that there are particular thoughts that cause anxiety, and these may be linked to and driven by your beliefs.

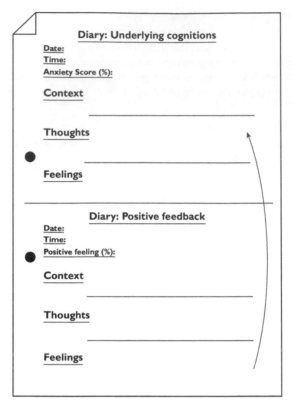

Figure 4.1 Diary: underlying cognitions

Keep a diary, to identify and monitor those thoughts that make you feel anxious, along with those that are more positive and empowering. Review and explore the nature of your underlying cognitions. See Appendix, Figure A.3.

Underlying cognitions

In normal life, we are not aware of the nature of the structural components that constitute our underlying cognitive world. We are just aware of the way that the world makes us feel. If we spend some effort (as we have done previously in this book), we may have started to access some of our conscious thoughts and thought processes, and perhaps we have tried to reframe them. We may, indeed, have spent some time trying to dissect out and consider some of our underlying beliefs (that may or may not be unhelpful to us). Now, we will try to explore further our underlying cognitions, in an attempt to gain a better understanding of why we feel so anxious in relation to the OSCE (see Exercise 4.1).

Behaviour and physiology

So far, we have documented our anxiety, put it in a context, and listed our thoughts and feelings. This is helpful, and will allow us to see patterns form and identify significant thoughts and contexts that trigger our anxiety. However, other key aspects of this cognitive model are the behaviours it induces and the physiological reactions it creates. Often, the resulting behaviour and physiological

EXERCISE 4.1 UNDERLYING COGNITIONS

A useful way to access and identify your underlying cognitions is to keep a diary of times when you feel anxious and overwhelmed by the examination, and try to identify what happened to trigger off this anxiety state. Usually, there is a particular thought that triggers a state of anxiety, and it would be very useful if you could make a note of this at the time. Over time, you will start to see patterns forming. You should also keep a record of instances in your life that challenge the underlying belief that you are a failure. Review this diary, and remind yourself why you are not a failure, and why you should pass the examination.

The objective of this exercise is to try to access your underlying cognitions, and to do so you must keep a record of emotionally charged times of anxiety. At such times, it is difficult to see objectively beyond the anxiety, but, if you look back, you may make more sense of what was happening cognitively. Also, you will be collecting evidence to challenge any underlying negative beliefs, such as, that you are a failure.

Recording

Label a pocket notepad diary 'underlying cognitions' (see Figure 4.1), and try to carry this with you at all times. This is an exercise that cannot be planned; you must collect the information as and when it presents itself. If you become anxious about the OSCE, or unusually anxious about other aspects of your life during preparation for your OSCE, make a note of the date and time in the notepad, and mark down the degree of your anxiety as a percentage score.

Under this, write 'context', and list the factual information surrounding the onset of the anxiety. This will include the location, who you were with, what was said, what you were doing, where you were going, what you were eating, what you noticed in the environment. You should fill in as much factual contextual detail as you can. Write enough so that you can recall exactly what was happening when you felt anxious. In that way, you will be able to reconstruct your memory of the anxiety later, when you are no longer feeling anxious.

Underneath your contextual facts, put a new heading: 'thoughts'. Here, you list what you were thinking at the time of the anxiety, and try to distil the thoughts down into their basic building blocks. If you were thinking about food, list exactly what food you were thinking about. If you were thinking about financial problems, write down the exact details of what money troubles popped into your mind.

Underneath your thoughts, put another heading: 'feelings'. Here, you capture what you were feeling. Try to describe the emotional content beyond just 'anxious'; you need to be capturing the essence of what you actually felt.

Repeat this every time you feel anxious, with each episode recorded on a new page. At the end of each day, or perhaps every few days, when you are not feeling anxious, you should review your diary. Aim to make at least one entry per day. Read through your records, and think about the contextual factors, the thoughts, and the feelings surrounding your anxiety. Try to remember exactly how it felt, and even though you don't feel anxious now, you should try to remember the nature and form of the anxiety. Does this make you feel anxious? If so, record this on a new page—list exactly as above, and carefully note the context, thoughts, and feelings.

When you review the records in a non-anxious state of mind, you need to try to identify the most important thought that occurred at the time of the anxiety. You will find that there is usually a more prominent thought—a thought that triggers your anxiety and makes you feel bad. Underline the most important thought with a red pen. Then, draw a line between this thought and the most significant feeling (recorded below) that it is linked to.

(continued)

EXERCISE 4.1 (CONTINUED)

By doing this exercise, you will start to get an insight into the thoughts that are making you feel anxious. Keep this diary going. The more that you can understand your underlying thought processes, the more in control of anxiety you can become. The diary will give you an insight into the type of underlying beliefs that you carry with you. Look for patterns in the nature of the anxiety-provoking circumstances, and the thoughts that occurred. What is the belief structure that links these anxiety-triggering thoughts? For example, if the triggering thoughts always tended to be linked to money and finances, you might realize that your underlying negative belief is that you will become bankrupt. Break down and record your underlying cognitive processes, look for patterns, and gain access to your underlying belief structure. Once you have identified your underlying beliefs, you can start to challenge them.

The second component of this exercise is to keep a record of those instances when you receive positive feedback and affirmation from patients and colleagues. This is the antidote to the poison of the anxiety. When you feel positive, make a record (as described previously), and score the positive feeling as a percentage. Under this, list the contextual factors, then the thoughts, then the feelings. These pages should look similar to the anxiety pages, although this time you are collecting positive experiences. Review the positive affirmation pages in the same way you reviewed the anxiety records: think about how you felt; underline the most significant thoughts; and link these to the most significant feelings listed below. By doing this, you are developing an antidote and cognitive strategy to counteract your anxiety.

Reflecting

Review your diary, both positive and negative. See how the negative thoughts differ from the positive thoughts, and how they are linked. You will probably find some similarities between these two different thought processes, though they make you feel very differently. Negative underlying cognitions and beliefs are reinforced by many things. Try to break this cycle of reinforcement. Analyse your underlying cognitive processes, highlight patterns, and actively think about the cognitive aspects of your anxiety at the time when you are most anxious. Identify your underlying beliefs and challenge them.

By doing this exercise, you have become an investigator of your own anxiety and mental state. You should take a step back and research your thoughts and feelings. You are observing your own anxiety; you are deconstructing it into its component parts. Observing anything changes the nature of that which is observed. In this way, you will change the nature of your anxiety. Pull off the shroud of secrecy and analytically assess the thing that has been causing you so much distress.

responses have an effect on the anxiety state itself, and they can also act as reinforcement to the underlying beliefs.

Previously, I have illustrated this cognitive model by telling you about the time I was mugged. Instantly after that trauma, I formed the underlying belief that I would be mugged again. This wasn't a conscious realization. I only realized this when subsequently reflecting on the situation with a colleague. This belief made me feel very anxious whenever I was outside, and resulted in a physiological reaction (increased heart rate, increased respiration rate, etc.), particularly when I felt unsafe. My anxiety led me to behave in a different way—I had lived on that road for eight years and never taken the bus (it was only a ten-minute walk), but I had started to use the bus. Travelling by bus relieved my anxiety and made me feel better. However, every time I took the bus, I actually was reinforcing the underlying belief that I would be mugged again. My behaviour was reducing my anxiety, but positively reinforcing my underlying unhelpful (and untested) cognitive processes and beliefs.

Now that you have made a diary of your anxiety (see Exercise 4.1), we can start to explore the findings in a more detailed way, taking into account your physiological state and your resulting behaviours. This will be very useful for a number of reasons. Firstly, you will develop a deeper understanding of the thought processes and behaviours associated with anxiety and beliefs, and this will allow you to start to challenge the underlying cognitive processes. Secondly, the problem with OSCE-related anxiety is often the actual physiological responses and behaviours themselves. So, starting to understand and get to grips with them is crucial as they can directly impact on your OSCE performance.

For example, anxiety can make a person's hands shake. We could try to explore that before the OSCE and aim to reduce it, by challenging the underlying beliefs that drive the anxiety state. Or, alternatively, we can continue to behave in a way that reduces our anxiety in the short term, neglecting and often reinforcing the underlying belief. However, what do we do then in the actual OSCE? If we feel anxious, get shaking hands, and relieve the anxiety in a way that won't be possible in the actual OSCE, then the anxiety and shaking hands will be back with a vengeance during the examination. If you relieve your anxiety by working hard on learning your content skills, then it will return in the examination because actually, you are not addressing the core reasons driving this. Likewise, any method you use to reduce anxiety in the short term (such as alcohol, distraction, or denial) is useless if you can't employ it in the actual OSCE.

For the sake of example, let us consider a candidate who has failed their OSCE, is feeling anxious, and noticed that their hands shook during their last attempt. That candidate will almost certainly feel less anxious if they delve into relearning their content skills, but at the next OSCE, their hands will still shake, perhaps more. Thinking about this in the theoretical construct of a cognitive model, the underlying cognition would be something like the candidate believing they will fail again. The physiological response is shaking hands. The shaking hands themselves reinforce the anxiety and also the underlying belief. The behaviour (of studying content skills) relieves anxiety but reinforces the underlying belief. Indeed, the person is working so hard on their content skills because they think if they don't, they will be a failure—so these things are explicitly linked. I hope you can see how a feedback loop can form easily, and how behaviours can act to perpetuate that loop. Breaking this loop isn't easy, but forming an understanding of its components can be very helpful, and, if you can visualize the components of your own anxiety feedback loop, then you can start to try to disrupt it.

Changing behaviour

It is very hard to change an underlying belief, although you can try to understand it and challenge it. It is impossible simply to deny your anxiety state, and dampening it (by alcohol, distraction, or denial) will only work in the short term. We are also unable to change our physiological responses; we can't use willpower to stop our hands shaking. These responses are beyond our conscious control. So how can we break this feedback loop? We can change our behaviours.

The way that we behave is driven by how we feel, and, in a cognitive model, the behaviour reinforces the underlying beliefs that drive the anxiety. We can change the way we behave. By doing this, we have gained access to the cognitive feedback model. Our behaviour is modifiable, and is, therefore, our access point for real change. However, this would only really work if you understood the theory behind this cognitive model, and appreciated the weight and impact associated with behavioural change. If I just happened to walk home because the bus was cancelled, I probably wouldn't have felt so differently, but because I made the choice to change my behaviour and walk home (against my natural instinct to get the bus and doing so in the knowledge that I would be feeling very anxious and expecting to be mugged), then when I *wasn't* mugged, it had real impact and therapeutic value.

You have kept a diary as suggested in Exercise 4.1, and have started to explore, dissect, and understand your underlying cognitive processes. You will now construct a cognitive model that takes your behaviours and physiological responses into account, and start to find ways of modifying your behaviours in an attempt to access the cognitive feedback loop and effect change (see Exercise 4.2).

EXERCISE 4.2 BREAKING THE CYCLE

1. At the top of a piece of paper, write down a significant anxiety-triggering thought as identified in Exercise 4.1 (see Figure 4.2). This is a thought that makes you feel anxious, or is linked to your anxiety state in a significant and meaningful way.
2. At the bottom of the page, make a note of the feelings that result from this thought (also identified in Exercise 4.1), with arrows from the thought to the feeling. The feeling must be directly linked to the thought. There may be more than one feeling for each thought.
3. On the left hand side of the page, half way down, make a note of the physiological responses that you've noticed occurring alongside the anxiety resulting specifically from this particular thought, with these particular feelings. Examples of this could be increased heart rate, tremor, hyperventilation.
4. On the right hand side of the page, half way down, note the behaviours that are linked to your thoughts, feelings, and physiological responses associated with the anxiety. What do you do typically when you feel this exact way? How did you act in the contextual example recorded in your diary (see Exercise 4.1)? Is there a pattern to your behaviours? Do you behave in a way that reduces your anxiety? For example, do you have a drink? Do you call a friend or watch television? Do you study? Do you think about something else? Do you go for a run? What *actually* do you do?
5. In the top left corner of the page, make a note of the contextual situation or trigger that resulted in the anxiety and the most significant thought (which should be listed in the 'context' section of Exercise 4.1). What happened to make you feel this way? Is there a pattern forming?
6. In the top right corner of the page, try to capture what you think the underlying belief is that drives and perpetuates this cycle. What is the underlying belief?

Once these areas have all been completed, you should draw arrows to make links between the different aspects of your anxiety. The thoughts already link to the feelings below (those overt links were made in Exercise 4.1), and so you should add the arrow accordingly. Feelings can also have an effect on our thoughts—so the arrow should go in both directions. Next, consider the feelings and how they make your body respond physiologically. Draw an arrow leading from the feelings to the physiological responses. Also, think about how your physiological responses can feed back and modify your behaviours—so this arrow also should go both ways. Now, think about how the thoughts lead to the behaviours. Think about that link, and the significance of it, and draw an arrow linking the thoughts to the behaviours. Draw an arrow from the triggers to the thoughts.

Physiological responses have a big effect on our behaviours, thoughts, and feelings, so you need arrows from here to all three areas. Indeed, a panic attack is an extreme example of this—a physiological response that makes you think you are dying, which exacerbates the physiological responses, and so on. Consider how your physiological responses change the way you think, feel, and behave.

Finally, the behaviours. These have a profound effect on emotions, physiological responses, and our thoughts, so draw an arrow to these three areas. The way that we behave is crucial

(continued)

EXERCISE 4.2 (CONTINUED)

and key in this process. Think about your behaviours, and consider the strength and significance of the links that you have just made between them and your thoughts, feelings, and physiological responses.

Carry out this exercise for all of your identified trigger thoughts. Are any patterns forming? Are there any repeated behaviours? You now have a visual representation of your anxiety, and this alone will deepen your appreciation of the links between thoughts, feelings, behaviours, and physiological responses.

The final stage of this exercise is to choose a behaviour and modify it in the context of experiencing the anxiety. If you notice that you have a drink of alcohol when you feel anxious, change that. If you watch television, stop doing that. Whatever the behaviour is, try to modify this in some way while you feel anxious. If modifying the behaviour makes you feel *worse*, then you know that the behaviour is linked to the anxiety state. In this way, you know that you are accessing the cognitive cycle.

By changing our behaviours, whilst understanding the significance of these behaviours in the context of a cognitive cycle, we can access this unhelpful cycle and work towards breaking it. It may take time, but you should make a conscious choice to modify your behaviours, and to live with the increased anxiety induced by that change. In doing so, you are breaking the cycle and stopping the reinforcement of the unhelpful underlying cognitive processes and beliefs that drive your anxiety state.

By embracing your anxiety, you are doing some psychological weightlifting; you are burning through the pain to get stronger.

Modifying your behaviours in this way should initially lead to an *increase* in anxiety. If it doesn't, then the behaviour is not sufficiently linked to the anxiety in the first place. Usually, your behaviours act to reduce anxiety in some way. So, by changing these behaviours, you will lose that comfortable reduction in anxiety. However, you will also stop the unwanted reinforcement of underlying cognitive processes and beliefs (see Exercise 4.2).

Outside help

If you feel overwhelmed by anxiety, then you should seek professional help. Psychological strategies would probably be a very useful treatment option, and your GP can advise you of what services are available for you. Sometimes, it can be helpful to have a way of snapping you back into an objective state of reality, distracting yourself from your anxiety. Some people use an elastic band on their wrist for this, and they literally snap the band against their wrist at times of anxiety. If you plan to try this, use it in study sessions, and get used to connecting the snap of the elastic band with regaining control and feeling less anxious. You may find it useful to discuss anxiety in your study group, thereby forming your own support group. It is often helpful just to air anxiety and think of it collectively, rather than suffering in solitary silence.

Some candidates will seek medication to help with their anxiety. This decision needs to be made in collaboration with your GP. If time permits, it would be better to explore psychological strategies before resorting to medication, but if medication is to be used, then the candidate must ensure that they do not use the tablets for the first time at the OSCE. Ideally, your study sessions should replicate exactly your body state in the actual OSCE. So, using medication just for the OSCE and not the study may not be advisable. Whilst I don't advise using medication, it is better to get your anxiety under control rather than being overwhelmed and paralysed by it in the OSCE.

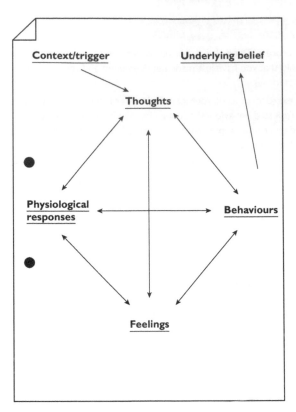

Figure 4.2 Breaking the cycle

Identify behaviours that you can modify, in order to disrupt the reinforcement of unhelpful underlying beliefs and cognitive processes. See Appendix, Figure A.4.

The main thing is that you should accept anxiety, and embrace it as an essential component of your preparation for this process. Use anxiety as it was intended—to enhance your performance.

Further reading

1. Gelder, M. G., Andreasen, N. C., López–Ibor Jr, J. J., and Geddes, J. (eds.) (2012). *The New Oxford Textbook of Psychiatry* (2nd edn). Oxford University Press, Oxford. (See sections 4.7 and 6.3.2, considering anxiety and its psychological treatment.)

CHAPTER 5

Confidence and self-belief

CONTENTS

Nurturing confidence

The previous chapters have helped us to consider our psychological baggage and unhelpful underlying beliefs and how these can be detrimental to your performance in the OSCE. We have spent effort in reframing these towards something healthier. We have swept the house clean and got rid of all the old junk—but now we must furnish our house with nice things that will make us feel happier and more confident. Unfortunately, our subconscious cannot be furnished easily with confidence and self-belief, and, whilst in this chapter we will consider the importance of confidence and the way that it affects our performance, we won't necessarily become genuinely more confident. We will, however, think about confidence in a slightly different way, and I will suggest ways to nurture your confidence and improve the conviction of your self-belief.

Physical 'tells'

Your degree of genuine confidence and self-belief shines out to your examiners: it is a physical 'tell', and you need to take control of it and use it as such (see Box 5.1).

BOX 5.1 'TELLS'

Imagine a poker player. A bad poker player will show their hand by giving away their physical tells; but a great player is aware of their tells, in control of them, and uses them to their advantage. A great poker player exudes confidence and self-assurance and belief when they need to, and can also fake fear and despair at will. This misleads the other players into either betting or folding: they are controlled by the 'tells'.

Of course, it might be great to be genuinely confident in every OSCE station, but the reality is that we are all human, and OSCE stations can go wrong. I would suggest that if you feel genuinely confident in every scenario, then perhaps you should be more careful and rethink your approach (see Chapter 2, 'Over-rehearsal' section). We should, instead, model ourselves on a great poker player, and use confidence as a 'tell' in the same way that they do. Confidence should be considered and applied—not too thickly (as over-confidence is worrying to examiners)—but applied nonetheless. You can appear more confident by: smiling; making good eye contact; with a firm handshake; and being calmly in control. Apply confidence deliberately.

I have just watched the 2013 men's tennis final at Wimbledon, and was struck by the importance of psychology in this game. Often, what makes a tennis player a champion is their ability to fight back from a position of 'failure', and indeed sometimes, a player's skill improves when their back is against the wall and they are fighting for survival. This is normal, and any of us, in any given situation, will focus usually more reserves and effort into a task when we are failing; our performance can be improved and augmented. Some sports players challenge themselves during a match to enable them to regain their edge. I'm thinking of a famous snooker player who changes to his weaker left hand to challenge himself more during important games. Unfortunately, when we are pushed to the edge, and are using all of our efforts and resources to improve our performance, this is usually written all over our faces. Watch a tennis player with their back against the wall, fighting for survival, and you can see the stress and fight very clearly in their body language—their 'tells'. In the OSCE, when we are stressed and are fighting to regain control of our performance in a particular challenging scenario, our body language will also tell that story. The difficulty with this is that, as a medical practitioner, we are judged partly by our external body language and composure, and so we can't afford to show our stress and anxiety. Indeed, a key objective is to be calm, collected, empathic, caring, and collaborative, even when we are putting all of our efforts into the content skills required for the task. Therefore, we must wear a mask of confidence and self-assurance, in the same way a poker player does. We don't have the luxury of the honesty that a tennis player has: we must hide our stress and fake our confidence. We must take control of our physical tells, and use them to our advantage.

Process skills

Our stress is illustrated to the examiner through the quality of our process skills, and so, we must think carefully about those non-technical skills and try to reduce our negative 'tells' to a bare minimum. For example: eye contact; body language; empathy; communication—all of these things can suffer when we are stressed, and if these aspects of our presentation suffer, then the examiner (and patient/actor) will get a poorer impression of us. A good practitioner maintains the quality of all of these non-technical aspects of their performance, and, sometimes, the non-technical aspects are more important than the technical 'content' that we are delivering. If we are discussing something difficult with a patient or their family, then it can be the case that the way we interact is just as, or more, important than the actual content. Or at least, if our interaction isn't successful and the patient/actor loses confidence in our abilities, the factually correct content may simply fall on deaf ears.

Whilst we can make efforts to minimize the deterioration of our physical tells, by optimizing our process skills, we must accept the fact that our internal emotional state will certainly leak out to a certain extent, and will be seen by the patient/actor and examiner. Our external tells and composure are significantly influenced by our confidence and self-belief, and if we can enter the OSCE station feeling calm, confident, and 'successful', then we will project a better external impression to those around us. Added to this is the phenomenon that we tend to feel more confident if we act more confidently. This is a self-fulfilling prophecy. So, whilst we can wear a mask of confidence, we must also try to improve our core internal state so that we feel more confident and believe that we are a success.

Dressing confidently

There are certain conventions as to what one should wear in an OSCE, and these are partly dependent on your particular specialty. However, it goes without saying that your clothes must be comfortable and familiar, but also must be smart enough to take you out of your comfort zone and make you feel confident and professional. You need to blend in with the other candidates, but also feel individual. You need to dress smartly (as though you were attending an interview) but, at the same time, remember that the OSCE is a hands-on demonstration of your day-to-day clinical skills. Therefore, you must dress in a way that would feel comfortable at work. By wearing very smart clothes that we wouldn't normally wear, we do feel more confident—but this is only a thin sheet of frail glass, easily cracked and broken by a stressful and challenging OSCE scenario. True confidence comes from knowing that you are behaving in exactly the same way that you would in a stressful situation at work.

Eye contact, body language, and speech

Always make good eye contact—this is essential. Try to smile, if that is appropriate. Be purposive in your movements and body language: if you are holding your hands together, you are doing it on purpose. Be in control of your posture and body language: soften your position if you need to (see Chapter 7). Your voice should be even, calm, and controlled at all times. Everything you say, and the tone in which you say it, needs to be purposive. You need to be fully in control of your external self—this is your body suit of confidence. You need to step into this body suit in every study session, indeed in every patient interaction between now and your OSCE.

Operate externally

Confidence gives the impression of internal strength, and should appear effortless. Many of the negative psychological aspects that spoil our OSCE performance are situated internally, and are exacerbated if we focus on our internal selves. To overcome these difficulties (as well as to follow the method described previously in this book), we must try to move away from such introspection and operate externally. Think less about yourself, and concentrate on the world around you. Focus your attention primarily on the patient/actor, but also consider the wider environmental perspective. Do not allow yourself to dwell internally—distract yourself with every word the patient/actor says, every movement, things around you. Focus on what is going on in the patient/actor's internal world. This takes priority over your own internal struggles. By operating externally, you can also apply, objectively, those physical tells that give the impression of confidence (good eye contact, posture, etc.).

Self-belief

If you are at the stage in your career of being able to attempt a particular OSCE, then I would suggest that you must believe that you are ready to pass that hurdle and move on in your chosen specialty. If you don't believe you are ready to pass, then perhaps you are not ready to attempt the examination. It is not enough to believe that you are a good and successful health practitioner—you must believe that you will be seen as such by the examiners in the OSCE. This can be a problem if you have already failed, and all of the previous chapters are relevant here.

Any negative baggage and beliefs need to be considered, reframed, and challenged. Use the previous exercises to do so. By taking away the negative, we allow the positive to flourish. If you believe that you are a good practitioner day-to-day, then you should believe that you can pass the OSCE. It is as simple as that. If there is something unhelpful blocking this link, for example, a belief that the

OSCE is a flawed examination, then you need to use the previous exercises to break down that blockage. Your belief in your abilities to perform well day-to-day should flood into your reserves of self-belief regarding the OSCE.

Further reading

1. Yeung, R. (2011). *Confidence: The Power to Take Control and Live the Life You Want*. Pearson Life, London. (This is one of many books available designed to build confidence.)

CHAPTER 6

Understanding OSCE construction

CONTENTS

OSCE development

We won't dwell on this, but I thought it might be useful to just reflect briefly on how OSCEs are developed, and thereby give you more of an insight into what is required for success.[1] Breaking down the OSCE is the main ethos of this book, but, conversely, it is useful to have a grasp of the component elements that were used to construct your OSCE. It's a bit like watching DVD extras to gain an insight into the film-making process: once you have seen how a particular scene was story-boarded, lit, and shot, the magic of the scene is broken and the technical aspects of the work can be appreciated. After this, new scenes can be broken down in an informed way and understood from a slightly different perspective.

An OSCE station is very much like a scene from a movie—including an actor (or a well-rehearsed real patient), a script, an audience (the examiner), and a clinical narrative (that you write as you go; see Chapter 13). The success or failure of the scene depends on your ability to play your part in this production, and you need to bring authenticity to the part. You are a health practitioner and you are acting in exactly the same way you would during a real patient encounter. This is a real-life simulation, in the same way that a movie scene simulates whatever it is depicting. If it doesn't seem real, then it won't work. So let us consider this scene, and how it was created. What is the purpose of the OSCE station? What is it testing? What does it strive to demonstrate to the audience (the examiner)? How can you play your part in this production?

Blueprinting and station development

The purpose of an OSCE is to test content from a core curriculum, and good content validity depends on accurate matching of the clinical skills tested with the required learning objectives and competencies of the curriculum. This is achieved by the use of a *blueprint* in OSCE examination design.[1] Whether planning a bank heist, rescuing a prisoner, or negotiating the hurdle of the OSCE, knowledge of the blueprint is essential. What is the map that was used by those constructing the bank, prison, or examination? If we can understand that map, then we have a chance of success. The blueprint is the underlying premise for an OSCE examination, and insight into this gives you more of an idea of what the examination actually is testing.

For this reason, I suggest that some basic knowledge about blueprinting and station development is very useful, especially when rehearsing pre-existing OSCE scenarios in your study group. Instead of getting lost in the specific content of an OSCE scenario, and spending effort memorizing what information is required for each one, you should consider the blueprint that was used to design this OSCE examination and the individual station development that helped test key elements of that blueprint. Think about the blueprint. What are the key skills being tested, and how do these map onto learning objectives from your core curriculum? Think about station development. How was this station designed to test key competencies and skills, and what were the building blocks?

If you break an examination down to its blueprint, instead of getting distracted by the specific information required in a particular station, you start to realize that blueprints appear again and again. The details change, but the skills linked to the core competencies are revisited time and time again. Once you can deconstruct an examination to its blueprint in a study session, you will have gained an improved insight into what the examination actually is testing overall.

Likewise, if you can see past the noise of the specific information required for a particular station you are rehearsing and instead concentrate on the key elemental building blocks that were used to map the clinical skills tested to the components of core curriculum, then you will naturally also start to gain an insight into the building blocks in the actual OSCE—and recognising the building blocks enables you to equip the skills needed to negotiate those blocks.

Building a blueprint

So what is blueprinting? When an OSCE examination is designed from scratch, the designer will first choose learning objectives from the core curriculum, and then make a decision regarding which domains of clinical skills are to be tested. The key aspect of the blueprint is that the learning objectives must map onto the clinical skills tested, and, usually, the educational elements are mapped onto one axis and elements of skills are mapped onto another. Using this blueprint, the OSCE examination can be suitably balanced and the appropriate range of different educational objectives can be achieved.

It is a useful exercise to make a list of the stations that appeared in your most recent OSCE examination and, for each scenario, extract the main objective from the core curriculum that was tested. These headings form your 'x' axis. Then, for the 'y' axis, use the main skills tested in the examination (for example: history; explanation; examination; procedures). Make a grid, and then fill in the key component that links the educational objective with the skill, from the stations in this particular examination. For example, they may have chosen to test the 'examination' skill with the 'gastrointestinal' (GI) system by use of an abdominal examination; and, perhaps, they tested the 'explanation' skill with the GI system by asking you to explain gastroscopy. This all sounds very obvious, but if you do this for the whole examination, you will see the blueprint they used to design that particular OSCE. Repeat this for a few more OSCE examinations and patterns will start to form. This is the value of deconstructing the examination, cutting through the trees to get an overall picture of the wood.

Developing a station—the construct

Next, we will consider individual station development. A newly designed station will start with a clear premise or *construct*, a clear statement of what it is testing. This construct will not be stated explicitly to the candidate of course. However, the examiners will see this—for you, as the candidate, identifying the construct is a significant step towards succeeding in the scenario. What is the underlying construct for this OSCE station? This can be worked out from old stations, and, whenever you practise a scenario, always try to establish a clear construct. By learning to identify the underlying construct in rehearsed scenarios, we can start to understand how a construct leads to the finished station, and thereby see through the gloss of a real-life OSCE station and into the underlying construct.

An OSCE station must include clear instructions (either written or verbal) for the candidate, so there is no ambiguity or confusion. If carefully read (or listened to), the instructions will tell all candidates exactly what to do. The instructions will not state explicitly the construct of the station, but, with practice, you can gain an insight into the nature of the underlying construct. Of course, never assume a particular construct. This could be very dangerous. One must always remain open-minded and ready to change course, but trying to identify the construct, rather than getting lost in the details, will be helpful. Try to see the wood, rather than getting lost in the trees. What are the needs of this patient/actor? What is the examiner looking for? Which skills need to be demonstrated that link to a core competency being tested in the station? What is the key?

Marking

There is a trend for OSCEs to be marked using global rating scales rather than a checklist approach, and generally, this is thought to be better for trainees as they become more experienced.[2,3] However, many of you will know, from the feedback sheets, that there is some inconsistency in this, and whilst the principle of global rating scales is sound, one should always be careful to cover all the bases. There are some checklist items that are essential, and we are all aware of those 'red flag' items in our own specialties. However, as a general rule, OSCE stations are designed to be marked with global rating scales, and, therefore, it is important to perform well globally in the scenario. It is not enough to recite a memorized list of pertinent questions. One must be led also by the verbal and non-verbal cues that the patient/actor delivers to you, and you must react accordingly.

References

1. Boursicot, K. A. M., Roberts, T. E., and Burdick, W. P. (2007). Structured assessments of clinical competence. *Understanding Medical Education*. Association for the Study of Medical Education, Edinburgh.
2. Cohen, R., Rothman, A. L., Poldre, P., and Ross, J. (1991). Validity and generalizability of global ratings in an objective structured clinical examination. *Academic Medicine*. **66**: 545–8.
3. Hodges, B. (2003). Analytic global OSCE ratings are sensitive to level of training. *Medical Education*. **37**: 1012–16.

Forming a connection

CONTENTS

Being empathic

Empathy is one of the core tenets of being not only a good practitioner but also a caring and sensitive human being. Empathy is an innate social skill that enables us to comfort a friend who has just received bad news, or a patient who is suffering inside. It lets us reach inside another person and connect with them on a very basic and primitive level. Empathy is a key process skill that enables and facilitates our human interaction and communication, and, here, we will consider the formation of our connection with the patient/actor in the OSCE.

Some trainees can project themselves empathically and form a connection very naturally; some find this more difficult. However, all need to consider the challenge of connecting with a patient/actor in a stressful OSCE station lasting several minutes. OSCE scenarios are artificial standardized tests of clinical skills that are time-limited and involve a noisy room, lots of stress, a patient/actor, and an examiner. We all know, going into the OSCE, that this is just a simulation and not real, but while we are in the scenario, with the patient/actor, we must connect and demonstrate empathy skills that are as sincere and robust as they would be if we were comforting our best friend about some bad news.

Emotional weight

Empathy is a social skill that is easy to spot and examine objectively. The examination of empathy is done partly by the feelings it invokes in the examiner, not just by the actual words that are said. You know this yourself. If you watch a badly acted play or film, then you feel nothing emotionally, but if you watch the same play acted well, those identical words can have incredible poignancy. Empathy is not the words themselves, but rather the *emotional weight* driving those words. To be truly empathic and form a connection, you need to really care. You need to care about the patient/actor, in this artificial situation, in a draughty hall with noise in the background and with bells going off every few minutes. It can't be just words, just an act—it needs to be *real*. This is a problem, because if we were investing truly in every single OSCE interaction, if we were empathizing genuinely and connecting on a human level, we would burn out and be emotionally exhausted after a couple of scenarios.

Often, a trainee will say that they are always empathic in a real consultation, but they find it hard to be empathic in an artificial OSCE station. However, once you have been a health practitioner for many years, you may find yourself on-call on a Saturday night, seeing your seventh patient in a busy A&E Department, with limited time, and feeling exhausted—under these circumstances, it is very hard to be naturally empathic. This is because we are only human and only have so much emotional energy to give. Also, this is a very difficult, emotionally challenging job. So, if we connected emotionally with every single real patient, we would soon get exhausted and would quickly burn out.

Empathy is a very useful hands-on skill for a practitioner, and is an extremely powerful way of allowing us to connect with, and quickly extract information from, strangers. So, in one sense, the OSCE is a very useful and realistic simulation of front-line clinical interactions, and, in order to be successful, we must utilize our empathy as an overt skill in the same way as we might use it successfully in A&E. In this chapter, we will start to dissect into and investigate empathy, in order to utilize it in our OSCE.

Body language and facial expression

Good empathy is much more than just words—to be truly and sincerely empathic (on tap) you need to employ your whole body and face in the activity. This, of course, comes naturally if you are comforting a close friend or family member over a coffee, but is not so easy to do when faced with a patient/actor and examiner in your OSCE. With a friend who has just confided in you with some painful news, you might put a hand onto theirs. Of course, you wouldn't do this to a patient/actor, but you might relax your body, drop your shoulders slightly, and soften your posture in a way that engenders warmth. Think about the non-intimate ways that you might react to a friend, and employ these in your OSCE rehearsal. If someone tells you something painful, you certainly shouldn't continue sitting straight upright as you were. Shifting your posture, in any way, is helpful, as it expresses non-verbally your acknowledgement of the painful interchange. If you can soften and relax your posture, you will make the person feel listened to, cared for, and at ease.

Any body language employed should be very subtle and barely noticeable. It is not about overt movements but, rather, subtle shifts in posture. The cinematic cliché is a head tilt when someone tells you something that is painful to them, and perhaps a subtle version of this might be effective. You need to try different ways of adjusting your posture when you are being empathic.

If a patient/actor is disclosing something painful, you need to be silent and let them speak, while at the same time prompting them and encouraging them to continue. You can do this by softening your posture; giving small, subtle nods and shakes of the head to acknowledge key points; and, perhaps, changing your posture in response to the information delivered. You can add in the odd gentle 'mmm' to encourage speech, but be careful not to speak while they are speaking. If they dry up, but you get the feeling that there is more, then you could coax them gently to continue with a couple of words, such as: 'I'm sorry...' or 'I understand...' Your body language can speak volumes in this situation. If you sit rigidly in silence, you will get nothing more; but if you sit in relaxed empathic silence, you will draw more out of them. Your relaxed empathic posture might be with shoulders slightly dipped, head slightly tilted, palms facing up (instead of down)—you are in a posture that is vulnerable and caring, rather than in a defensive professional posture that protects you. Whatever your posture, it must feel very natural to you and can't be forced.

In your OSCE, most of the focus will be on your face. The examiner and patient/actor will be looking mainly at your face, and your facial expressions are a very powerful way of showing warmth, caring, and compassion. It is worth videoing your own facial expressions during rehearsal and seeing the way you utilize your face as you deliver and listen to information. Empathic speech without the corresponding facial expressions is unconvincing and lacks impact. If you are told something that is painful, your face must react. It is not just about saying the right thing in response: you must use your facial expressions to convey your acknowledgement of the painful information. If you are comforting a patient/actor, or telling them that you are 'very sorry to hear that', you must match your facial expressions to the words. This, of course, comes naturally in real life, but it needs to be actively practised for use in the artificial OSCE scenarios.

Also, remember that non-technical skills such as facial expressions may be forgotten whilst trying to negotiate a difficult task under pressure. Therefore, you must practise these skills. Rehearse emphasizing your facial expressions in everyday life and during OSCE practice. Video your face and work on improving your expressions. Watch movies and take note of facial expressions. Then copy these. Once you have worked on emphasizing your expressions, try to scale them down, so that they are subtle and natural.

Distilling empathy

I will now suggest a way to try to dissect empathy and extract the essence of this essential social (and examination) skill (see Exercise 7.1). Considering and breaking empathy down in this way will increase our subjective understanding and appreciation of this very natural and amorphous non-technical skill, and we will attempt to glean some empathy triggers that may be useful to employ.

This is an exercise designed to deconstruct, distil, and package a complex, multifaceted process skill into something that is retrievable and accessible to you in your OSCE. Later in this book, we will

---

EXERCISE 7.1 DISSECTING AND REPACKAGING EMPATHY

There are moments in life when we feel particularly emotionally connected to others. This might happen with a friend, a partner, a family member, or even whilst watching a good movie or reading a moving novel. The objective of this exercise is to collect these moments, write them down, and extract the memories, thought content, and feelings from the emotionally charged moments. By doing this, we will try to break down the cognitive processes that occurred during these emotional moments, understand them, and utilize the pertinent thoughts and memories in the artificial OSCE scenario in order to trigger the emotional content of the very real, previously experienced moments.

Buy another notebook and dedicate this one to empathy (see Figure 7.1). Each page will be a record of an emotionally charged moment, when you felt moved and connected to another person. If you need source material, then re-watch any movie you have found emotionally moving in the past. I suggest that you collect these real-life moments over the weeks after your written papers, and capture them as accurately as you can.

1. At the top of the page, write a single sentence that encapsulates the emotional moment. A statement that captures the emotion—concise and poignant, but detailed enough to be understood by a friend reading it.
2. Under this sentence, draw a line, and in the second section write down how you felt during this poignant moment. Describe your feelings using individual words or short phrases. Be as detailed as you can in capturing your feelings. Then, draw a line under this section.
3. Below this, in the third section, make a note of the context: time, date, where you were, and who you were with. If you were at dinner, make a note of the food and, ideally, anything particularly striking you recollect, such as the smells and the colour of the tablecloth. If you were at the cinema, make a note of the people sitting around you. This third section of the page needs to include enough detail so that you can accurately recall the emotional content, and link the emotional content and feelings to the little subtle

---

(continued)

EXERCISE 7.1 (CONTINUED)

details and memories. Think about how the small details are connected to the emotion on a cognitive level. Link the details with the emotion and feelings. Draw a line under this section.

4. In the fourth section, make a note of the thoughts that were going through your head at the time. For example, if you were watching a movie where a person dies with their partner at the bedside, you might think how sad it was that the partner was left alone, how touching the moment was, how sad the death was, how it affected the family left behind, etc. Capture as many thoughts as you can. Consider how the thoughts are linked to the emotion written at the top of the page and the feelings you described. Recall the thoughts, and link them to the feelings and the details. Draw a line under this section.

5. Divide the fifth section into three columns. Label the left column, 'feelings'; the middle, 'context'; and the right column, 'thoughts'.

6. In the left column, write down the most important words that describe your feelings. In the middle, write a list of single words that capture the most vivid details you remember, such as: 'red', 'garlic', 'restaurant'. In the right column, make a short list of single words, dissected from the thoughts written in the section above, that capture the essence of the thought—for example: 'bedside', 'family', 'alone'. Look at the words you have written in the three columns and think about how each word links to the feelings, context, and thoughts in the sections above, and then think about how the single words link with the emotional content in the moment captured by the sentence at the top of the page. Make a robust cognitive link between each word and the emotional content.

7. Draw a line under the three lists, and use the space at the bottom of the page to choose the most powerful and poignant word from the 'feelings' column and the 'context' column, and the most powerful word from the 'thoughts' column. Write only one word in each column. So, the emotional moment will have been distilled down to one single word that captures a feeling, one that captures a detail connected to that moment, and one single word that captures the most powerful thought. Think about these three words, and make the connection between them and the sections above, ultimately connecting them to the emotion listed at the top.

8. Now, choose the single strongest word and copy it below—this is your trigger for the emotional content. You may, for example, have chosen the word 'red'. You will think of 'red' in the context of this particular emotional moment, and you will have formed a cognitive pathway between this word and the emotional feeling from the moment.

Do this for every emotional occasion, every moving moment in a film, every intense conversation, and every time you connect with another person (whether a real person or fictional character). By doing this, you will be deconstructing empathy, and you will be dissecting out and contextualizing the pertinent thought and emotional content. This will help you to understand your empathy, and you may see patterns starting to form. At the very least, you will be trying actively to dissect empathy and understand it on a cognitive level.

Now you have a way to trigger genuine emotional feelings. When you are in your OSCE, you can use these trigger words to access the emotional content in a very real and practical way. So, if you reach a point when the patient/actor starts crying in this very artificial situation, instead of just saying 'I'm sorry, that must be very difficult for you', you can access some emotional content to drive the empathic statements. An empathic statement only works if it is delivered with sincerity. By using these triggers to previously experienced emotionally charged moments, you can use those moments to add weight to your delivery and comments.

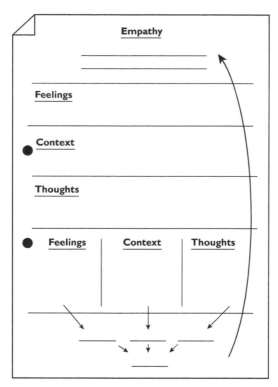

Figure 7.1 Dissecting and repackaging empathy

Record, deconstruct, and explore your subjective experience of empathy. Distil the essence of your empathy and develop empathy 'triggers' to employ in your OSCE. See Appendix, Figure A.5.

use a modified version of this exercise to do exactly the same with your clinical skills. This will allow you to access quickly the clinical skills that you need. In this way, you will build and utilize your skills toolkit. If you practise this exercise a few times now, using 'empathy', you will refine your technique and find it much easier later in the book. Packaging something as complex, subjectively qualitative, and difficult to distil as 'empathy' is much more challenging than using the same technique to package a pragmatic clinical skill. So, if you practise this now, with empathy, you will package your clinical skills into your skills toolkit with ease later in this book.

Empathy tone

Empathy should be a passive skill, ever present during your OSCE stations, and modulated in intensity according to requirements. Never discard empathy as being redundant—it is always a useful skill, even in the most practical of scenarios. Empathy is the buffer you use to dampen and protect the interface between yourself and the patient/actor. By *empathy tone*, I mean the degree to which you modulate your performance by increasing the degree of your empathy. In this way, think of empathy as having a control slider, that can move between zero and ten.

If your empathy control slider is set at zero, then you have zero empathy tone, and you are interacting with the patient/actor in a very pragmatic, cold, paternalistic, and non-caring way. You should never have your empathy tone set at zero. Even if you are performing life support or a central line on a mannequin, you should still never have your empathy tone set at zero. Never have your slider set below one—one is the absolute minimum. In that way, no matter what the situation, you will come across as a caring health practitioner, who puts the needs of the patient paramount in any situation.

With your empathy tone set on the maximum at ten, you are the most empathic you can possibly be. Never operate at a ten. You need to save ten for that extra burst of speed and manoeuvrability that might just get you and your motorbike out of an unexpected motorway pile-up ahead. No matter how upset a patient/actor becomes in the OSCE, there is always headroom for a bit more anguish. If you are empathizing to the max with a crying patient, and then they tell you that their child was killed last week, you have nowhere to go: you need to save some empathy headroom.

This may sound strange, but, actually, the examiner is assessing your ability to connect with and collaborate emotionally with a patient, and if the patient/actor delivers you even more anguish, then you need to demonstrate clearly to the examiner that you have modulated your engagement accordingly. You do this by increasing the control slider of your empathy tone. So, when a patient/actor challenges you with something painful or upsetting for them, then you can demonstrate to the examiner that you have recognized this, that you understand the need for a more caring approach, and can increase the tone of your empathy (thereby becoming overtly more gentle and caring in the eyes of an observer).

With regards to your starting empathy tone, set this at a comfortable mid-point, perhaps a three or four. In this way, you start the interview gently but confidently, open and caring, and giving the patient/actor and examiner the impression that you are there to listen and understand. Don't start too empathic: you need to be able to turn up your empathy tone if the scenario requires it; and, likewise, to turn it down if some positivity and containment is required.

Subtle paternalism

It is sometimes important to turn down the tone of your empathy, and move from a gentle, caring, understanding standpoint to something more positive and subtly paternalistic. An example of this would be when a patient/actor is telling how difficult their situation is, and, whilst you start by showing understanding in a gentle empathic way, you then shift into a more positive standpoint and instil hope by suggesting a new treatment strategy.

To do this, you must start with your empathy tone set at about five, collaborate in the patient/actor's difficulties, and demonstrate caring and understanding Then, pull your slider down to three and introduce a new treatment strategy in a more positive, hopeful, and enthusiastic way. In this way, the subtle paternalism pulls you slightly away from the patient, and puts you in a more positive and objective standpoint, towards which you can draw the patient with gentle coaxing and clear concise reasoning. Of course, a new hopeful treatment strategy must be very carefully explained, and this often will form a significant part of the OSCE task.

With regards to paternalism, in my opinion, the only time you should be paternalistic is when you need to *contain* a patient's anxiety and instil hope and optimism. In this way, you are addressing the needs of the patient. You certainly shouldn't be operating in a paternalistic way as a rule, since, if you do that, you will lose the useful impact of adding in a sprinkle of paternalism if the situation needs some lift and containment. Remember, though, that there is a fine line between expressing a confident, containing, subtly paternalistic attitude, and appearing paternalistic and uncaring to an observer. If you treat the patient with utmost respect and autonomy, then you can afford to add in a sprinkle of paternalism for therapeutic effect. However, do so with caution and in a purposeful way.

Candidates from overseas

Candidates from overseas, who have learnt their trade in a culture that demands a more paternalistic approach, will find this adjustment of empathy tone difficult. If, culturally, your patients demand and expect paternalism, then your core people skills will be instilled with this. If you were not paternalistic, then your patients would not respect you, and you would thereby lose a crucial and powerful thera-peutic effect. If you are paternalistic, you will not collaborate and connect with the patient/actor, and doing so is essential in the OSCE. So, you must confront this, and work on your instilled core paternal-ism. Reconstruct a core process skills set and perspective that is more collaborative and inclusive.

Mirroring

The empathy you deliver in your OSCE station needs to be matched to the degree of emotional intensity you are confronted with, and this is most easily achieved with subtle *mirroring*. As a general rule, your empathy tone should be set slightly higher than the patient/actor's degree of distress. That is to say, if they are speaking gently, you should be speaking a little more gently; if they speak even quieter and softer, then so do you.

Your whole delivery, including verbal and non-verbal communication, should mirror the patient/actor to a certain extent. To enable this, you must listen very carefully and pick up on all of the verbal and non-verbal cues that are delivered to you. Everything that the patient/actor says and does is either scripted or expected by the examiner—you must not miss anything. You shouldn't react necessarily to absolutely everything, but you should notice everything (see Box 7.1).

BOX 7.1 MIRRORING AND RESPONDING

If you are performing an abdominal examination and the patient/actor winces, you must react accordingly by verbally acknowledging their discomfort, modifying your technique, and then checking that it is okay to continue. This is essential and basic OSCE tuition. Actually, all you are doing is mirroring your performance to the patient/actor and modulating your delivery in accordance with what the scenario requires. So, if during a cardiac history, a patient coughs and looks away as though upset for a moment, you should pick up on it—you shouldn't just plough on blindly with your checklist of questions. It may be that a particularly stressful and relevant event has occurred, and the patient/actor is directing you to that paragraph in the script. At the very least, you will demonstrate an innate understanding of the patient/actor's needs, and you will appear caring and empathic. Therefore, in any OSCE scenario, always mir-ror your presentation, to a certain extent, in response to theirs.

If a patient/actor slumps their shoulders, then you need to modify your sitting position accordingly. The importance isn't so much in your actual position, but more that you are reacting to their change in stance. If the patient/actor shouts, then you need to raise your voice slightly (to be heard, and also to have sufficient impact and authority). If a patient/actor sobs and their speech is so quiet to be almost inaudible, you need to stop and speak more quietly. Just reflect their presentation. Actually, this is a very useful way of gaining trust and, ultimately, getting more information in a timely fashion.

'Tells'

An advantage of mirroring body language is evident in candidates who have anxiety 'tells' in their own body language, for example: picking their fingers; playing with their hair; general fidgeting. You need to appear calm and relaxed during your OSCE, and if you have 'tells', you need to be aware of them. You can try to master them by incorporating your own body language, consciously, into your performance (see also Chapter 5). Body language needs to be rehearsed and honed, and you should practise adjusting your own subtle non-verbal cues in accordance with what is delivered to you by the patient/actor. Of course, body language has to be absolutely second nature and require no mental effort during the OSCE. Therefore, these innate passive skills need to be practised and perfected during rehearsal. Although it is agonizing to watch back, it is very useful to video yourself rehearsing and, afterwards, analyse your body language objectively.

Learning to listen

Listening to patients is what we do. It is our job. We listen to the way that they express their physical state and symptoms, and we translate that into a context and structure that we can communicate, understand, and treat. Listening is not just paying attention to every specific word spoken; it is also making note of the way that those words are delivered, and includes paying close attention to other more subtle forms of communication. Body language can communicate a lot about a person's internal state (worth remembering when you think about your own internal state and body language during this exam). We must make a mental note of every glance, every twitch, every normal and abnormal movement. Listening is an essential component of truly connecting with the patient/actor.

Assessing and understanding a patient is a subtle art that takes knowledge and experience to master, and it is much more than just registering the words that are spoken. However, listening and making note of every single word is absolutely essential as a baseline in any assessment, and even more so in the OSCE when the patient is either actually an actor with a script, or a patient who has probably volunteered to help in this particular simulation many times before. Every word the patient/actor says is important, and not a single word can be missed.

You must practise listening to every word in your study group. This sounds obvious, but when I have facilitated study groups, it is usually clearly apparent that words are missed in almost every rehearsal. This is because a candidate tends to be more concerned with what they will be asking next, rather than with what the patient/actor actually is saying. You must listen to and process every word that your colleague says in the study group (see Exercise 7.2).

EXERCISE 7.2 **LEARNING TO LISTEN**

Rehearse your listening skills, in your study group, by adding in extra words and phrases for your colleagues when you are the patient/actor—these are potential *clues*. Each time a station is run, drop in novel words or phrases amongst the established narrative of the scenario. For example, you could be explaining how you have found yourself spending more money in the last two weeks, then drop in that it has been very warm lately. Did they respond? Did they follow the potential clue? Feeling warm could possibly indicate a thyroid problem. You need listen to every clue, and try not to miss anything.

You should try to add a new clue to every scenario you run. The clue may lead to nothing, and the words may just be added to see if the 'practitioner' hears them. However, your clue may lead onto something more important, that the practitioner would need to follow in order to be successful in the scenario. The observer should also listen carefully and make a note of the clue, and how the practitioner responded to it. Did the response address this new unmet need adequately or follow the lead successfully? Was the clue ignored?

Feedback the hit rate for clues, and, hopefully, the number of missed words and unheard clues should reduce collectively as the study sessions progress.

Essentials

Connecting with a patient/actor and demonstrating good empathy skills is not just something you learn to do: it is important that you try to instil a sense of genuine emotional weight to your empathic statements, along with the appropriate corresponding body language. However, here are a few basic pointers and tips that might be helpful for you to consider:

1. A patient/actor is a human being. Listen to the patient, and try to react to them in the same way that you would react to a friend who has just told you their bad news. This has to be natural. If the patient/actor tells you: 'My son was killed three weeks ago', you need to react with a flavour of the way you would if a friend gave you this devastating news. Of course, you won't be quite as emotionally charged with a patient/actor (for example, you wouldn't cry with them or embrace them), but they are a human being, and you need to add a strong flavour of the emotional content and support you would deliver to a friend in the same situation.

2. Never speak when the patient/actor is speaking, and if a patient/actor starts crying, stop speaking. Do not, *under any circumstances*, speak over a weeping actor—not until you have been caring, empathic, and asked permission to continue. If the actor starts crying, pause. Then say, gently: 'I'm very sorry.' Then pause again. Then say: 'I know this is very hard, can we continue?' Do not continue the interview until you have acknowledged their distress in a caring, genuine way, and then been given their permission to continue. Do not continue as though nothing has happened.

3. Listen to everything the patient/actor communicates and react in a human way. We are all people. If you treat the patient/actor as a human being, then you will probably, very naturally, demonstrate empathy skills. Just be kind, gentle, and caring, while at the same time moving the interview forwards and covering the information you need. Success depends on getting the balance right between your caring, gentle, empathic approach and your control of the interview.

4. If the patient/actor is upset or shuts down, be gentle. If you are feeling the pressure of time and frustrated that the patient is not saying what you need to hear, be ever more gentle. The more frustrated and stressed you feel, the more gentle you should be.

5. Use pauses—pauses in an OSCE station lasting several minutes are very impressive and very powerful. If the patient is finding it difficult, pause, and seek permission to continue. Pause. Ask them if they understand. Pause. Ask them if they want to know anything else. What are their concerns or anxieties? What are their needs?

6. Be relaxed. This will make the patient/actor feel at ease, and the examiner feel more confident in your abilities. Be gentle. Speak slowly and clearly.

Forming a connection is a core skill that must be second nature to any candidate in an OSCE. The best empathy is emotionally driven, and it is useful to develop ways in which to access emotional memories and content. I have suggested a way this might be done. Empathy should not need to be thought about in the actual exam: it should already be there as a passive skill, and your tonic state needs to be one of being caring, calm, and understanding. Please devote thought and time to forming a spontaneously robust and meaningful connection with your patient/actor, and take this very seriously, since it will make your life a lot easier in your OSCE and will be a useful skill for the future.

Further reading

1. Baron–Cohen, S. (2012). *Zero Degrees of Empathy: A New Theory of Human Cruelty and Kindness*. Penguin Books, London. (Useful if you want to think more about human connection and empathy.)

CHAPTER 8

Rehearsal

CONTENTS

The need to rehearse

It is not without a sense of irony that after saying how important it is in the OSCE to be *real* and not to act, you now have a chapter titled *rehearsal*. This is not actually a contradiction. We work in a job where we need constantly to elicit and deliver sensitive information, and to do that effectively, we need to be warm and empathic and caring. We need to do this just as efficiently even when we are rushed, stressed, tired, unhappy, and perhaps are trying to deal with a much more urgent and pressing matter at the same time. So how do we do that? We *act*. Acting is a part of being a good health practitioner. That is not to say that we don't really care, but it is inevitable that there will be times when we have to give the impression of caring and connecting when we simply don't have the reserves to be so.

Acting is an important part of being a professional health practitioner. Our jobs are challenging, and we need to project an image to the public. Acting protects us as health workers. It allows us to leave work at work, and assume our true selves at home. When placing a cannula for the first time, the medical student or junior doctor is absolutely terrified, but they must try to project the image of an experienced expert for the sake of the patient. This is acting. A more senior health practitioner may be rather timid and softly spoken, but they must project the image of a confident, firm team leader when directing a resuscitation attempt. When a trainee surgeon and consultant discuss a difficult operation using local anaesthetic, they need to project calmness in any discourse so the wide-awake patient is not unduly distressed. There are many situations, many real scenarios, when a health practitioner needs to act. Acting is an essential skill for us all.

Even the greatest, most naturalistic actors rehearse, and for us, good rehearsal is essential because we need to perform on a very pressured, noisy, stressful, expensive, and important stage. We can't afford to have a bad performance in any one of our fleeting appearances, and the way we do that is by rehearsing.

Your rehearsal must strive to reconcile the contradiction between the simulated patient being both a 'patient' and 'actor' at the same time. Rehearsal needs to refine and standardize your responses and interactions, so that you will behave the same way to a real patient in a busy A&E Department as you would a patient/actor in the OSCE, and also as you would a colleague in your study group.

In doing so, you will be a better practitioner in all of these environments, and good group rehearsal strategies can result in a change in clinical practice that will stay with you throughout your career.

Rehearsal strategies

A child who has to learn and memorize a list of information for the first time will usually start rehearsing the information by reading and re-reading the list. They might read it out loud, and some would find that more helpful than others. They might make a visual representation of the list, by writing it in a particular way. They might annotate the list, mentally, in order to remember it. As we develop and progress through our education, we each discover our own best way of learning and rehearsal, and, as this method becomes more sophisticated, it tends to become more of an internalized mental process. It is worth reflecting on your own formative rehearsal strategies, as these can give you an insight into the complex, sophisticated, internal way that you memorize things now.

The information required for an OSCE has usually been mostly already attained. There may be more content skills to learn and refine, but learning the factual knowledge is not usually the aspect of the OSCE that makes it so challenging. It is translating that knowledge into seamless and effective clinical practice that creates difficulty. Rehearsal strategies for the OSCE should concentrate on the translation of knowledge into clinical skills, and this is best done in a group. Each group member will have their own optimal way of rehearsing, but you must form a collective, collaborative rehearsal strategy that works for all.

A rich contextual tapestry

A collaborative rehearsal strategy can be very effective, since the collective can contribute to the rich tapestry of information available for the group to learn and rehearse. During our formative years, our rehearsal strategies will have incorporated different contextual elements in order to make learning more effective, and as we develop this skill, we will incorporate, unconsciously, a combination of visual, auditory, and cognitive techniques to maximize our subsequent recall. In a group, each member can contribute to this rich contextual tapestry and offer different dimensional aspects of the material to be learnt. This might take the form of anecdotes and analogies, pictorial representations, jokes, lists, mnemonics—a number of different perspectives that will improve your rehearsal strategy.

Raw study material

To be successful in your OSCE, you need to know all the stations that have been used previously. This is not in order to learn them by heart, but to have a good idea about the way the College uses the curriculum to construct the examination blueprint. So, each study group member should investigate a particular year of previous OSCE examinations to see what came up. This can be done easily by trawling through the different specialty OSCE forums online. Once a list has been made of the actual stations in each examination, this can be correlated to the masses of written and online material for these particular scenarios. It is possible, with some research, to find detailed model answers for most of the scenarios that have presented themselves in the different examination sittings.

However, in the group, you should not get too hung up on rehearsing the specific content and model answers. It is my view that the most important thing to rehearse is the broad type of scenario that is examined and the skills needed to negotiate that scenario's pitfalls, not the particular answers given in that particular station. Candidates often prepare for the OSCE in the wrong way. You shouldn't be focussing on the information required for a particular station; you should be building generic skills and strategies that would work in *any* station. Just use the stations that have already come up in previous OSCEs as tools for study and self-improvement.

The whole performance

Good rehearsal technique is essential for the OSCE, and this needs to be developed and worked on. There are no set rules, but it is better to add in as many contextual elements into the rehearsal process as possible, and give the group a rich tapestry of information to work with. Imagine actors rehearsing for a movie scene or play. They already know the words, and they are rehearsing at a higher level in order to transmit emotion to the audience. That is your task. It is not enough merely to know the facts—you must rehearse the whole performance.

A good health practitioner is also a good actor, even when they genuinely care for their patient. Acting is our defensive shield that keeps us strong and compassionate in the face of emotional exhaustion, and allows us to pour inexhaustible comfort and compassion into every single patient interaction. So, whilst the OSCE may seem artificial, it forces us, actually, to develop and rehearse crucial clinical skills and psychological defences that will help us for the rest of our clinical careers.

The whole performance

CHAPTER 9

Studying in a group

CONTENTS

Rationale for study groups

The OSCE examination is a simulation of a real clinical experience, and your group study needs to recreate this as closely as possible. The more realistic the simulation, the more useful and powerful it is. You can't recreate the actual cubicles and stressful environment, but you can match other elements quite closely—for example: exact station timings, bell rings, ambient noise in the background. We will consider some important aspects of group study here.

Group membership

This needs to be friendly yet brutal. The members of a group need to click, and not all people click in this situation. If a person isn't right for this particular group, then they will certainly be right for a different one. If a person comes into the group and is more aggressive and competitive than the rest, then they need to be in a more competitive group. They simply won't benefit from your group, and will merely be getting an instant confidence boost by being a bully. They will not grow and develop; they need to be studying with like-minded bullies.

Learning to be critical

Feedback is an important part of the learning process, and your study group should develop ways of providing feedback that is useful and *formative*. Feedback should inform and improve your future performance. The feedback element of any study group is one of the reasons that the group membership needs to be right. At the end of the day, we are all competing with each other in this examination, but the study group should be a team that is internally non-competitive. All the group members need genuinely to care that the others pass, and you should go into the rehearsal process and examination with that ethos powering you. You don't need to be friends initially, but you definitely need to become friendly, and a successful study group will probably result in a small group that will be friends for a long time to come.

Once you all trust each other and have been studying together, you can start to criticize each other's performance. However, this needs to be careful and gentle. You don't always need to say good things, and, indeed, this is most unhelpful. Useful criticism points out the cracks and weaknesses in a performance and suggests ways that a person might improve, but it should do so very carefully. Try not to get too hung up on only highlighting the information that wasn't delivered. It might be useful to say if major things were missed, but a study group isn't merely a forum in which to learn scenarios. The criticism should focus on wider issues such as performance and empathy. Even if you watch a video recording of yourself, you won't spot your body language as well as others can. So, you could gently criticize body language and suggest ways of improvement.

The study group needs to be reflective in nature. In that way, it should be a safe place where people feel confident enough to air their insecurities and deficiencies. It is not a place where some are better than others. All are equal in their goals, treatment, and respect.

Group ownership

When a scenario is run in the group, the group as a whole should spend some time objectively thinking about how it went and how it would have played out ideally. The group should assume *ownership* of the scenario. It should not just be a critique of the performers themselves. Of course, participants may want and expect feedback, but it is important that the group, as a whole, first reflect on the *facts* of the scenario. Doing this allows open and objective criticism of how managing the scenario could be improved, without any particular person feeling inadequate. The group needs to work through the scenario as it played out, objectively describing what actually happened, and think of ways to improve the performance of the group as a whole.

If a particular person asks for feedback on their performance then this can be given, but it needs to be given carefully. Don't pander to a person's ego, and be wary of saying anything too critical as that person's confidence could easily be knocked. It is safest to learn, as a group, a technique for keeping criticism objective and descriptive. From this, a particular person can draw experience and implicit feedback of their own performance. The more you use this technique as a group, the more adept you will all become in gathering your own feedback.

Personal feedback

If a person really wants some more personal feedback on their performance, then, as a general rule, try to give them a 'feedback sandwich'—one positive criticism for every negative criticism, followed by a further positive criticism or comment (positive, negative, positive). Personal feedback can be very useful, but it should be given carefully and as objectively as possible. If you decide to give more personal feedback, then it is a good idea to ask the person who just performed the scenario to feedback first. This allows them to identify good and bad points first, and may avoid an observer needing to raise a negative point since it has already been covered.

After rehearsal, even the most hardened candidate will feel vulnerable. Be sensitive to this and be gentle with your immediate feedback. In time, you will develop a trust and understanding within the group that will allow more brutal criticism, but remember that the closer you are to the examination, the less able you are to modify and modulate your core responses and behaviours, so it becomes more redundant to give harsh, potentially confidence-damaging criticism. Like everything, successful criticism is a fine balance. A study group that provides useful formative feedback and criticism is much more powerful than a study group that glosses over this. So, it is a skill worth developing.

Separate the facts from the feelings

As a general rule, don't mix facts with feelings. Separate out your group's objective opinion of how the scenario should best be done, and don't involve feelings of 'how did I do?' or 'how could I improve?'. Once the group has covered the facts of the scenario and established the model answer, then it can consider more personal feedback and the feelings of the person who just performed for the group. In this way, the group takes ownership of the facts *before* carefully considering the feelings of the performer. When facts and feelings are mixed, it is harder to extract the useful learning points without potentially upsetting the performer or just concentrating on their needs. The needs of the group are paramount and, in this way, every single scenario rehearsal is useful for all group members.

Assigning roles

Using previous OSCE stations as raw material, the study group sets a timer and each member takes it in turns to be both 'patient/actor' and 'health practitioner' in the task, trying to be as genuine and emotive as possible in both roles. Other members of the group are observers, and should each observe a defined aspect of the performance (for example, content and process skills). Try to keep the scenarios active and fluid, rather than passive and static. I think that it is better to repeat the same station for all the group members rather than plough on relentlessly through all the possible stations. Your performance needs to be modelled and refined, and that is more difficult if you keep changing the scenario every time (see Chapter 10).

The patient/actor is in a strong position to inform the group how the candidate made them feel. Some group members may not appreciate the value of playing the role of the patient/actor, but this role is crucial. Indeed, in some OSCEs, there is a growing trend for patient/actors to contribute towards the marking of a station. Being the patient/actor gives you a good insight into how well the health practitioner is performing, and informs your own subsequent performance in the practitioner role. It also gets you used to acting—an essential skill for the OSCE.

The observers in the group are in a good position to give formative feedback. One person should focus on the content skills, but rather than getting hung up on the specific questions that might have been asked or the steps of a physical examination, think more about where the practitioner's line of investigation was going. Was this clear? Were they listening? Were they altering course depending on the patient/actor? Did they miss anything significant? The feedback should be along the lines of this—major headings rather than the small print. With regards to informing future performance, the feedback should be looking at the big picture. This person certainly shouldn't be saying 'You didn't ask X, Y, and Z...', although I know from observing study groups that this is often the main focus of feedback. Try not to get lost in the content. Content should be reviewed individually, outside of the study group.

One person in the group should be thinking about process skills, such as: question style (open and closed); non-verbal forms of communication (both from the practitioner's performance and those that may have been missed in the patient/actor's performance); empathy; body language. This second observer can be much more specific and detailed in the formative feedback they deliver, and this is perhaps the most important feedback.

Remember that the timing of the scenarios is critical. OSCEs are time-limited, and the group needs to get used to the feel and pace of the scenario in real time. All scenarios must be executed fluently within the correct time frame; not rushed, but brisk enough to cover all the required points. Be strict with the timings, and if there is a one-minute warning bell in your OSCE, then recreate that in the study session.

Be a team player

There is an inherent positive karma in being a team player and providing selfless, effective, empowering, formative feedback to others. You learn lots by helping others, and the best way of improving your own assessment skills is by trying to refine those of another person. It is useful for all candidates to get used to being scrutinized and judged by others, and helpful to get an idea of what others think about you. However, this needs to be done skilfully and compassionately. Keep your study group safe.

Post-session objective analysis

At the end of each study session, it is useful to think about the skills you have learnt as a group, and which further skills you need to cover. Think about where the study sessions need to go in order to cover the core curriculum, and where you would like to go next. Try to categorize your new-found skills in a more generic way, and discuss how you might use the skills in other types of scenario. You might be able to remember real encounters when you used a skill similar to one extracted in the study session, or perhaps you can think of real clinical examples that could have benefited from such skills. Try to attach real memories and experiences to the simulations and extracted skills. This will add weight and authenticity to the skills set you are developing as a group, and will contribute to the rich contextual tapestry you are all creating.

Post-session feelings

Once you have spent some time discussing the session in a descriptive and objective way, it might be useful to think, as a group, how you are *feeling*. A study group is a very useful space in which to talk about feelings pertaining to the examination, and it is very helpful to air, with your colleagues, any anxieties you may have. However, set boundaries for this discussion, and don't let the feelings bleed into the more objective talk of the mechanics of the session and scenarios. Anxiety regarding the examination and preparation process needs to be packaged into a safe place after the study session, and shouldn't be allowed to contaminate the rest of the session. With such boundaries, the good work done in the study session will be more useful, and the discussion of feelings after the session will have more power.

Try to package the caring, supportive aspect of the group wholly into your period of protected time at the end of the session, and be consistent with your future management of this. A supportive group setting benefits from consistency, and this allows the psychological setting to be nurturing and containing. This time at the end is precious, and whilst you will not be reducing your collective anxiety by working on the content skills during this time, you will be addressing the equally important psychological needs of the group.

Modelling

CONTENTS

Diagnostic edge

The more familiar you are with the OSCE stations that tend to arise, the more disadvantaged you can become. This is because as you become comfortable, you tend to lose your diagnostic and investigative edge. If you were a detective investigating a bizarre and unusual scene in a strange location, you would undoubtedly spot more clues than if you were in your own living room investigating who it was that had lost the remote control. In the first scenario, your adrenaline would fine-tune your senses into acute instruments, and no noise or smell would go unnoticed. In the second scenario, you would just look under the couch where the remote usually is. So, in this chapter, we will consider the value of *modelling* an OSCE scenario, and we will start to introduce subtle changes to a station that the group takes it in turn to rehearse, in order to make a familiar scenario more unusual. We will work towards heightening our diagnostic edge.

A modelling strategy

Repeat the same scenario within the study group several times (to allow everyone to try once). Each time the scenario is played out, something should be changed: the scenario should be active and fluid. By modifying the scenario and seeing how the candidate reacts to this modification, you will start to learn, as a group, how small changes affect the performance dynamics. Moving from one station, straight to the next, doesn't allow you to change the scenario in very subtle (but perhaps significant) ways. So, repeat the scenarios, to make them ever more unusual, novel, active, and challenging.

Modifying the scenario, as it moves around the group, will allow you to practise being fluid in your responses, and, sometimes, these changes may alter the direction of your investigation completely. You need to be able to think on your feet, particularly in a familiar scenario. There is really no point in practising a particular station and knowing exactly what to do, because you are likely to fall foul of the OSCE when a subtle modification is introduced. You need to adapt your investigation and approach according to the specific patient/actor and whatever they may say. In this way, if you come across a familiar scenario in which you need to assess abdominal pain, then you will be the candidate that spots the underlying rare problem, rather than the candidate that misses it. It is much better to walk out of the OSCE saying 'Oh no, that was a disaster, I only spotted the *xyz* in the last two minutes...', than saying 'That was great. At least one station I knew came up, and I gave a model performance...'

The following is an example of a generic OSCE scenario I have found useful when facilitating OSCE workshops. It allows fluidity as it moves around the group, because the scenario really can go anywhere. Of course, you will use a scenario appropriate for your specialty and profession, but Exercise 10.1 demonstrates how a basic scenario can be modelled within the study group.

EXERCISE 10.1 MODELLING

In your study group, the first person to be the patient/actor makes up a scenario: in this example, you are a female patient on a medical ward who wishes to have a termination of a pregnancy. That is all the information the health practitioner has, and they must assess the patient within the OSCE time frame. Run the scenario. The patient/actor must have in mind some facts about the nature of the request for a termination, but they will be prompted to answer questions (and, therefore, think of the answers) when the practitioner asks them.

After the initial scenario cycle has finished, the first observer in the group will feed back on content skills. They will mention any significant areas of investigation that were not covered, and will tell the group where they thought the lines of investigation were going. The second observer will comment on the process skills, questioning style and non-verbal communication, including empathy. As the second observer, view the interaction as you would view a film—think about the emotional responses and whether or not they had sufficient impact.

By going through this process as a group, you will have created a scenario, and from now on, the existing narrative of the scenario will be expanded on. For example, if the patient/actor mentioned they already had two children, this becomes a narrative fact of the scenario. As a group, you have started to create a station from scratch, and the narrative will be further enriched with subsequent run-throughs.

The whole point of the modelling is to model the group performance in the scenario. However, you do that by modelling the actual station components. By adding to, and refining, the narrative of the scenario, you make it both more complex and more challenging. You are literally building a brand new, complex, clinical scenario from nothing. In the process, you will be learning how the elements of the scenarios work together, and will, thereby, be starting to appreciate how other novel stations can be deconstructed.

So, the scenario moves round to the next person (from patient/actor to observer one, not to the practitioner role). In the next cycle, the same scenario runs, but this time, the patient/actor refines it in some way. For example, they may have been raped. (This may not have been asked during the first run-through, and could be prompted by the practitioner role in the rehearsal.) Once this traumatic past has been created, it becomes a new fact in this narrative you have created together. The patient/actor should also try to add in a 'wild card'. For example, they could say that they are worried about an inherited disease in the family, or perhaps they are desperate for the termination but they face family or religious opposition to this.

Go through the process of feedback, and cycle the scenario around the group. Build on the scenario. Add in emotive elements: for example, her son may have just died four weeks previously. Model the group's empathic response to this, as this new narrative fact in the scenario works its way around the table. Add in risk elements: for example, she has small children at home. Explore and expand on the risk issues: for example, she has been feeling violent

---

(continued)

towards her children. Add in some past medical history: perhaps she has been advised to terminate for medical reasons but doesn't want to do so.

The scenario may totally change direction as it moves around the table. What was a straight-forward assessment may quickly transform into a very sinister and complex clinical scenario. The value of adapting and refining the scenario from scratch, within the group, is that it teaches you how the components of a complex scenario work together, and it allows you to model your approach to investigation and empathy as the scenario is slowly refined and modelled from person to person.

Once the scenario has run a few times, or perhaps more if it is getting sinister and interesting, it is useful to write it down as a group. Write your own patient/actor instructions, and try to capture the scenario you created. When you read through the scenario, you will remember all the subtle things you learnt during the session. Annotate the notes with your own comments to jog your memory.

Finally, compare your scenario with an earlier one in the OSCE, and see how yours would have fitted into a previous blueprint of the examination. How well does your scenario match the core curriculum and content skills that have been tested before? You will really start to get a deeper understanding of OSCE construction by building a new, complex scenario, and comparing this to previous stations, whilst considering where it would sit in the context of a previous OSCE blueprint; and, also, by thinking about how the core curriculum and content skills link up. This deeper understanding will allow you to deconstruct, mentally, novel OSCE scenarios, and then apply the appropriate tools, extracted from your skills toolkit. Break the OSCE down, and apply whatever process and content skills are required to solve each component of this complex clinical challenge.

It is possible to model using previous OSCE scenarios, but it is better to take a known scenario and strip out all of the factual knowledge. It is important to add in contextual facts yourself, and then add to, and refine, the information as the scenario moves around the group. I personally think it is pointless to waste valuable study time trying to memorize previous patient/actor instructions—leave that to the professionals. We are health practitioners, and so we know what would make a scenario challenging and interesting. Inventing the details speeds up the study group, and OSCE station construction is a very useful skill to develop.

Modelling ourselves

Now you have a modelling template for your group, you can use that to model and refine your performance and approach. Just as the scenario has been formed and enriched with complexity and subtlety by the group, so should your performances be moulded and improved. As the scenario moves fluidly around the group, your individual responses and performances will also be refined and improved fluidly. This works well for both content and process skills.

Using video

It can be very unpleasant to watch oneself in a video recording, especially in the company of a group of people. Indeed, it can be excruciating and humiliating, and can make you feel a lot more self-conscious than you already did. However, it is an extremely powerful way to really see yourself as the world sees you. It can improve self-awareness, and, with this information, you can start to model your performance. I would recommend that you try to incorporate video recording into your study at least once, to see how you feel. With video, you can identify problems with your posture and body language in a way that others could not communicate to you. You need to see the problems for yourself. Ideally, you should use video several times, and note any improvement in the general way that you conduct yourself during the scenarios.

CHAPTER 11

Build your skills toolkit, part 1: getting started

Introduction to your skills toolkit

We will now consider building a skills toolkit to keep in our metaphorical back pocket. When you require a tool, for any given situation, you will reach in and deftly extract what you need. You will not be walking into an OSCE station with tools already in your hands; you will be walking in with fresh eyes and with your hands unburdened. If you walk into a familiar scenario with tools at the ready, you will be less able to pick the tool you actually need. In this chapter, we will start to transform our content and process skills into a more generic, modular, and transferrable form. In this way, we will be able to apply those skills in new and novel scenarios, and thereby be equipped to face any scenario.

From context-specific to modular, transferrable skills

Each clinical skill may be useful in many situations, and you need to categorize a skill in its most basic form. Don't think of a skill or strategy just in association with the particular station, sub-specialty, or systemic examination in which you learnt it. You should consider the clinical skills that you learn to be modular, transferrable, and adaptable to various different scenarios, as opposed to viewing each station as a separate entity to be mastered. Reframing your clinical skills into a more generic form is the first step in building your own skills toolkit.

When you rehearse an OSCE station in your study group, take a step back and consider what the scenario is testing. How do the clinical skills tested map onto the core curriculum? What is the underlying construct? What are they actually testing? How does this station sit in the context of the OSCE examination blueprint as a whole? Answer these questions in their most basic form, and don't get lost in the details—see the wood, don't get lost in the trees. What are the basic building blocks that were used to construct this scenario? Think of each scenario as a modular structural entity, and see beyond the specific facts and into the design elements.

When you develop clinical skills that are successful in your study group, break down and repackage those skills into their most basic form, and then practise their use in other contexts and scenarios. Consider how your new generic skills were useful in negotiating the hurdles you faced from the building blocks used to create the scenario. Think about how the basic clinical skills complement those basic structural elements used by the OSCE designers. This is the level at which you should be operating. Look beneath the surface of the specific station, and beyond the actual content required for success. You are operating on a different level, and you are building a collection of tools that you can use to negotiate whatever the OSCE designer throws at you.

A skills toolkit is very personal, and if you made a list and gave it to a colleague, it probably wouldn't be useful to them. The skills need to be packaged into the kit in a context that has meaning to you. I was told, very early in my medical training, that if you just read about a particular illness, you may remember it, but if you can match an illness to a face, perhaps the face of the first patient you came across with this illness, you will never forget it. Skills need to be given a context and a face. In this way, they are more powerful and more easily retrieved and utilized. Try to contextualize all your tools in the toolkit in this way. No skill should just be read in a book and then filed into the kit. Each skill should be rehearsed and refined, before being filed away into your toolkit for use in the OSCE.

Each station is a puzzle for you to solve. With every rehearsed scenario, you should be developing basic generic skills that can be employed in a variety of different stations. Don't get bogged down in the specifics of a given station; see beyond its noise and bustle. Examine the blueprint and design principles, think about the underlying OSCE construct, consider how the clinical skills tested map onto the core curriculum, refine the content and process skills, categorize them and file them away for future use.

Building your toolkit

So how do you actually build this skills toolkit? I have written a few exercises to illustrate this process, but the mechanism of building your own toolkit is very personal and specific to you. How you actually build your toolkit will depend on several different factors, not least of which is the very individual way in which you have developed your own rehearsal strategies over the years. Some people rehearse using auditory cues; some find it helpful to visualize information; some prefer to add anecdotal details in order to maximize their recall. As I suggested earlier, your rehearsal and recall should ideally employ a rich tapestry of auditory, visual, and cognitive cues. This provides the best way of learning and recalling process and content information. Whilst you do need to find your own method of building your toolkit, Exercise 11.1 illustrates the process of reframing a context-specific skill into a more modular and transferrable form.

EXERCISE 11.1 FILING YOUR SKILLS—INTRODUCTION

We will start with a skill needed for every single OSCE scenario—your introduction. When you approach the patient/actor, you must introduce yourself, but this shouldn't be totally stock and rigid. You might be more gentle in your introduction if you were seeing someone to break bad news, than you would if you were about to conduct a physical examination. A person on the cusp of hearing bad news needs a very gentle approach, whereas you might choose a more straightforward, professional approach with a person who is about to let you examine them. Your introduction should also include a request for permission to perform the interview or examination. So, practise your introduction in different styles. However, you must always remember to give your name clearly, and tell them what you do.

In your study sessions, you will notice that, as novice OSCE candidates, we tend to introduce ourselves in exactly the same way every time. If you find yourself doing that, you should question it. Your introduction should vary according to the task at hand, even if it only varies in the degree of empathy tone applied to your speech cadence. Rehearse different styles of introduction, and refine your style depending on the type of scenario.

(continued)

EXERCISE 11.1 (CONTINUED)

Break your introductions down to three basic types: an introduction for a physical examination; a history-taking version; and one for breaking bad news. Choose one of these three basic types for each scenario you rehearse. So, it wouldn't matter what you were examining, you would have a more straightforward introduction ready for a physical examination.

Next, you need to categorize the three types of introduction in a way that is useful to you. This might be writing them down, or speaking about them out loud, or perhaps mentally attaching them to a real-life clinical experience or shared clinical anecdote. The variety is endless, and you should select contextual elements from the tapestry created in your study group to help you to categorize the introduction types in a way that allows easy recall.

When you next practise a scenario, select the appropriate introduction from your toolkit by imagining your chosen contextual elements, and then apply the skill. Imagine the skill as a distinct object within your toolkit, and think about the way you retrieved it from your categorized filing system. Think about how the skills lie within the toolkit; visualize your filing system as a whole. Overtly think about the way you extracted the introduction that you applied, and imagine re-filing the skill for future use.

Familiarize yourself with your toolkit, and picture it in whatever way works for you. It could be as a filing cabinet or a utility belt, a computer filing system or a box of filed cards. The important thing is to separate out the introduction types from the specific scenarios, and file them individually. Then, you can retrieve them as and when you need, in any station.

Exercise 11.2 is another example to illustrate the process of taking a context-specific skill set, and reframing it into a more modular and transferrable form.

EXERCISE 11.2 FILING YOUR SKILLS—PHYSICAL EXAMINATION

Consider your physical examination skills, and the way that they have been learnt and rehearsed. You should be adept and fluent in all the body system examinations, and perhaps you have rehearsed integrating some of the examinations together. However, examiners may throw in a new station that does not consist of a well-rehearsed system examination. Consider facing an OSCE station you weren't expecting, such as: 'examine this foot'. A colleague of mine had this station in their MRCP OSCE, but was not expecting it, since feet are rarely the focus of MRCP stations.

Consider the body system examinations that include the foot, and think about which of these may be relevant in this unusual OSCE scenario. The clinical skills required to perform the system examinations are actually collections of well-rehearsed skills, and these need to be broken down and filed separately.

Divide all of your physical examination systems up into the component parts, and, along with the clinical skills, consider the diagnostic and investigative value of each part. Using the foot as an example, you might need to draw elements from orthopaedic, neurological, rheumatological, vascular, or even dermatological examinations. Practise formulating a differential diagnosis based on investigative findings retrieved from the selected components. Use this to contextualize the diagnostic weight and significance of the components.

Now, you have a collection of clinical skills extracted from the physical examinations of several body systems, and you understand the diagnostic and investigative weight and impact

(continued)

EXERCISE 11.2 (CONTINUED)

of these skills. The next task is to categorize these skills in a generic form, and file them into your skills toolkit for future use. They will not be just reintegrated into the body systems you extracted them from. Rather, they will be individually categorized and separately filed into your toolkit. This is the key step in building your own toolkit.

As before, categorize the skills in a way that is useful to you. Select contextual elements from the tapestry created by your study group to help you to categorize the skills for easy recall. Visualize the skills within your toolkit, and reflect on the way you filed them into your categorized filing system. Imagine your filing system as a whole. Perhaps write this down, or design a visual representation of your filing system? Perhaps the skills are colour coded, or have symbols denoting their purpose? Overtly visualize the way you filed the skills, and imagine extracting them again in the future.

You can see how filing the skills in this way could be a useful approach to tackle any unexpected request in the OSCE. You might want to practise this as an exercise in your study group, by setting a physical examination task that would not usually arise in your OSCE to each group member, and seeing whether they can respond by applying elements from their existing skills toolkit.

Dissecting and linking to contextual elements

Earlier in this book, we considered empathy, and I described a method of extracting and distilling empathic content from emotionally charged moments in life. I gave an example of how you could try to trigger yourself into feeling an aspect of the emotion you experienced during the emotionally charged moment, by deconstructing the thoughts, feelings, and contextual elements surrounding that experience. When we dissect into an amorphous, emotionally charged moment, and extract thoughts, feelings, and contextual elements, we can distil these down to powerful triggers for utilization in the OSCE.

We will use a similar technique now. Emotionally charged moments are very hard to break down, and, if you have already tried to do that, then you will find it much easier now to break down a clinical skill. A clinical skill (either process or content) may be simple or more complex, and, whatever its form, its purpose is to negotiate specific pitfalls in the OSCE. A clinical skill demonstrates your competency to the examiner and is usually pragmatic in nature: it fulfils its specific role and is, by and large, devoid of feeling, emotion, and context. If there were a context, it would usually just be linked to the situation where that skill was learnt and previously applied (although, of course, we have already been working hard to extract skills from their specific learnt context). We will now try to package our modular skills in a new way, using a contextual element drawn from the rich tapestry created in our study group (see Exercise 11.3).

EXERCISE 11.3 DISSECTING AND REPACKAGING CLINICAL SKILLS

In our OSCE preparation, and indeed our clinical training and daily work, we have accumulated and developed a wealth of clinical skills. These are the tools that enable us to function as successful health practitioners. The object of this exercise is to categorize and reframe these skills by: writing them down; dissecting into the thoughts and feelings linked to the skill; and assigning contextual elements that can be cognitively linked to the skill. By doing this, we will try to break down the cognitive processes associated with a particular skill, understand them, add in contextual elements, distil these down, and utilize the most pertinent thoughts, feelings,

(continued)

EXERCISE 11.3 (CONTINUED)

and contextual features in novel OSCE scenarios in order to trigger the memory of the skill. We will, in effect, be breaking the skill down in a way that can be easily filed and retrieved from our skills toolkit.

Buy another notebook and dedicate this one to clinical skills (see Figure 11.1). Each page will be a record of a clinical skill.

1. At the top of the page, write a single sentence that captures the pragmatic, clinical skill. Alongside this statement, assign a contextual emotive or evocative element. You have now linked the contextual element to that skill. The skill should be clearly stated and linked to a contextual element that is concise, poignant, but detailed enough to be understood by a friend reading it.

   The contextual element may be associated with the first time you ever encountered the need for this skill in real life (for example, a particular clinical scenario or patient), or it may be something that was discussed during a study session (an anecdote or even a joke). The contextual link needs to be evocative in some way, and has to be something you can feel or visualize. The context needs to be powerful. It may be something real, or just something that made the study group laugh. If you can't think of anything contextual, then make something up. Think of a patient or a scenario where this skill may be essential. Perhaps think of a movie, and how this skill might be portrayed dramatically.

   Linking the clinical skill with a strong, evocative, contextual element is essential. In the example I gave earlier in this chapter (your introduction to a patient), I suggested that you consider three different introductions. Thinking of one of those—for example, the gentle introduction to break bad news—the contextual link can be very powerful indeed. We have all encountered difficult situations where we had to break bad news, and we have all experienced how powerful and evocative those situations can be. Think of the most powerful scenario when you had to break bad news: that is your contextual link for that particular introduction skill. Capture the skill, and concisely describe the powerful, evocative, contextual-linked element. For the physical examination introduction, think of a physical examination that really sticks out in your mind. Was it awkward? Pressured in some way? This is the linked contextual element.

   If you have been able to link your pragmatic clinical skill to an evocative contextual element, then you have done most of the hard work. If you are just learning clinical skills in the context of previous OSCE stations, then you are wasting the potential of these clinical skills. You should reframe the skills, and link them to something more powerful and evocative. Take them away from the context in which they were learnt in your OSCE study, and reframe them into something more powerful and poignant to you.

   Under this sentence, draw a line.

2. In the second section, write down how you actually felt during this poignant evocative moment. Describe your feelings using individual words or short phrases. Be as detailed as you can in capturing your feelings. Draw a line under this section.

3. Below this, you should consider the details that establish the context written at the top of the page. Make a note of the specific factual elements that spring to mind when you consider this evocative, poignant scenario. When you broke the bad news, where were you? At what stage of your career were you? At which hospital did you work? What did the family say? How did they look at you? Did they cry? Were they angry? This third section of the page needs to include enough detail so that you can accurately recall the contextual element already noted, and link the context and subsequent feelings to the little, subtle, factual details and memories. Draw a line under this.

(continued)

EXERCISE 11.3 **(CONTINUED)**

4. In the fourth section, make a note of the thoughts that were going through your head at the time. For example, if you were delivering bad news at the bedside, you might think how touching the moment was, how sad the death was, how it affected the family left behind, etc. Write as many thoughts as you can. Recall the thoughts, and think about how they are linked to the context written at the top of the page and the feelings you described. Draw a line under this.

5. Divide the fifth section on the page into three columns. Label the left column, 'feelings'; the middle, 'context'; and the right column, 'thoughts'.

6. In the left column, write down the most important words that sum up your feelings. In the middle, write a list of single words that capture the most vivid contextual details you remember. In the right column, make a short list of single words, dissected from the thoughts written in the section above, that portray the essence of the thought.

7. Look at the words you have written in the three columns, and think about how each word links to the feelings, context, and thoughts in the sections above. Then, think about how the single words link into the evocative contextual element and clinical skill captured in the sentence at the top of the page. Make a robust cognitive link between each word and the evocative contextual element.

8. Draw a line under the three lists, and use the space at the bottom of the page to choose the most powerful and poignant word from the left 'feelings' column and the middle 'context' column, and the most powerful word from the 'thought' column. Write only one word in each column. So, the clinical skill and linked contextual element will have been distilled down to one single word that captures a feeling, one that captures a detail connected to that moment, and one single word that captures the most powerful thought. Think about these three words, and make the connection between them and the sections above, ultimately connecting them to the skill and context listed at the top.

9. Now, choose the single strongest word and copy it below—is your trigger for the clinical skill. You may have chosen the word 'sad'. You will think of 'sad' in the context of this particular clinical skill and linked contextual element, and you will have formed a cognitive pathway between this word and the clinical skill.

Do this for every clinical skill. In this way, you will be deconstructing your clinical skills and dissecting out and contextualizing the pertinent thoughts and emotional content. This will help you to reframe and categorize the clinical skills, and will allow you to easily file and retrieve those skills from your toolkit.

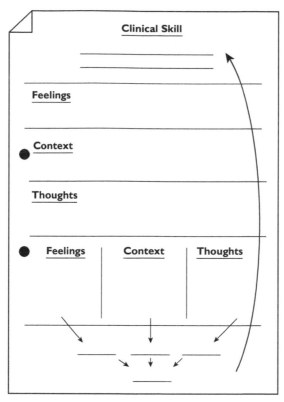

Figure 11.1 Dissecting and repackaging clinical skills

Repackage your modular clinical skills by linking them to emotive contextual elements.
Deconstruct and distil the essence of these linked modular skills, and develop skill 'triggers' to
employ in your OSCE. See Appendix, Figure A.6.

CHAPTER 12

Build your skills toolkit, part 2: general aspects

Generic OSCE themes

Over the next few chapters, we will consider an array of generic OSCE themes that are useful in many different scenarios, and I will suggest some strategies and solutions in each of these basic areas. In doing so, I hope to provide you with a generic strategic approach for each theme—a starting point from which you can develop your own modular and transferrable clinical skill sets. I have chosen themes that tend to include a degree of process skill in their successful negotiation, and I have tried to provide you with a way of moving forwards in each of these areas. We will draw this all together when we consider generic strategies later in this book (Chapter 16). In this chapter, we will first consider some of the more general aspects of your interaction with the patient/actor, using collections of tools that can be employed in most OSCE scenarios.

Seeking permission

A core principle of any assessment in the OSCE (or in real life) is that you have permission to conduct the assessment. You must have the patient/actor's permission *at all times*. Don't forget this, because asking for permission to continue is a very powerful way of restarting a stalled interview. I'll talk about this later, but, for now, we need to get started by establishing consent. We have to ask the patient/actor if it is okay for us to speak to or examine them. They may not want to speak to you. This could be because they are sick of waiting around in A&E and they just want to leave. Perhaps their impatience is driven by underlying pain? Whatever the reason, you need to establish the interview by seeking permission to start.

If the patient/actor says 'No', then you can't just trundle on with your assessment. This will look very bad to the examiner, and you will get nothing from the patient/actor. So, you must convince the patient/actor that it is in their interest to allow the assessment to occur. Do this by being progressively firmer (in your speech content, not tone) and more persuasive (though no less gentle, in fact more gentle), if you need to be. However you must be in control at all times. Try to prod them gently (metaphorically speaking) from all angles, rather than prodding in the same spot. You have to get to the core of why they don't want to interact with you. If there isn't time for this, you need to normalize the interaction and make them realize that you, and/or their family, are concerned. Explain that you would like to see if there is any way you could help.

If they are reluctant to speak to you because they are not 'ill', and perhaps are in denial about the possibility of a serious or rare illness, then you could reframe your concern by referring to other, more obvious and easier to explain, parts of the body. For example, use the analogy of a broken arm. Tell them that if they had broken their arm, they would need a plaster cast for it to heal. Everyone understands this, and even the most stubborn patient/actor must concede to that point. Their illness is no different, and if they are damaged or broken, they need to be fixed, in the same way as a bone needs to be fixed. Reframe their rare or serious illness into something that they are more able to understand and deal with.

If you are on a surgical ward and are seeing a post-operative patient with abdominal pain, the patient may be frustrated or anxious and may not want to tell the whole story to you again. Even in this case though, you can normalize the interaction by telling them that it is routine, a formality, for surgical patients to be followed up in this way. Contain their anxiety, and try to get to the bottom of their frustration. Normalize the encounter. If the patient has been brought in by a family member, you can say the family is concerned; or you can say that you are concerned. Make the patient understand that you are worried about them, and that you want to help (see Box 12.1).

BOX 12.1 A GENTLE APPROACH

In my OSCE, I came across a nihilistically depressed patient/actor who said nothing and didn't look at me for a couple of minutes after my introduction. Sometimes, you just need to try and try—different approaches from different angles. A general rule that I have mentioned previously in this book is that the more stressed you feel, the more gentle you should be. The longer a patient won't speak to you, the more and more gentle you should be, as you become more and more persuasive (and also probably more and more anxious yourself). Being gentle is the key: you can't force consent.

Starting open

Open questions, such as 'how are you feeling?', are more general, less challenging, and easier for the patient/actor to answer in a variety of ways. Open questions allow you to cast a wide net and sift for nuggets of gold. Closed questions, such as 'are you in pain?', are more specific, often more dissecting, can be more challenging, and are not as good for screening wider history points. As a general rule, you should always start your assessment with open questions, and then close the questions down as you delve deeper or if the patient/actor is not divulging what you need. The examiner will expect you to move from open to closed questions.

'Open to closed' is always the way you should investigate, but this approach is wider than just the actual questions. You need to approach the scenario with new eyes and a totally open mind, with no prejudices or preconceptions. Starting with a *panoramic view*, you should then adapt your generic strategy depending on what comes up. Start very open, and only close down your approach and become more specific when you are following a thread of investigation. You don't need to know what you are going to be doing before you actually sit down in the station, and appreciating this fact is very liberating. There is no point in feeling anxious in your circuit queue, or whilst reading any instructions outside the station. You decide how to steer your ship once you are in the actual scenario. You must focus all of your energy into these few minutes, and forget everything outside of this station.

The stalled scenario

This can happen in the OSCE, and the principle and tools required for restarting are similar to those used in seeking permission. If the patient becomes angry and shuts down, or becomes tearful, or finds it too painful—you need to reset the interview and get things rolling again by re-establishing consent. This is a very useful tool. If at any time in the interview things become difficult, then you can ask permission to continue. You can also use this if the assessment stalls because of you. If your mind goes blank, reset everything by re-establishing consent and start again from the ground up.

Being structured and understood

You are only a good communicator if what you are communicating is in bite-sized chunks that can be easily understood by the patient/actor (and, of course, the examiner). In some ways, this is a passive skill, because our communications should always be structured like this. However, it is a skill that you need to be aware of and that regularly needs to be actively employed to punctuate your OSCE engagement—even if you are in full flow and feel rushed against the clock. You should only be asking or telling the patient/actor as much as they can take in.

If you were writing an essay or book, you would use paragraphs and headings to break up the prose and make it more readable. It is the same in an OSCE: make sure you are regularly giving a heading in bold typeface, a *signpost*, and ensure that you are making it very clear to the listeners that you are starting a new section. Make it easy for them, and for you. Pause regularly, and ask them if they understand. Ask if they want more information. Seek permission to move on.

It is rather like doing a driving test. You want the examiner to notice that you are looking in the mirror. It is no use after the test, when you have failed because the examiner says you didn't check the mirror, telling him that you did actually look in the mirror. He needs to see you look in the mirror. So, when you do look, you give an exaggerated head movement that the examiner will definitely notice. It is the same here. When you are interacting with a patient/actor, make sure the examiner knows, by telling them, that you are now going to speak about side-effects of a medication.

The more rushed you feel, the more you should force yourself to pause regularly and split your speech up into chunks. Make it very clear what you are going to talk about next. If you really are rushed, then you will find that your investigation or explanation is actually much more efficient if you make that extra effort to punctuate it and split it into easy chunks. I said earlier that the more stressed you feel, the more calm and gentle you should be. It is the same with this: the more rushed you feel, the more you should be splitting your speech into 'signposted' chunks. Also, consider that during the actual OSCE, adrenaline will make your speech faster and denser. So, make huge efforts to break your speech into chunks that are easy to understand.

Illusion of structure

Learn how to generate an *illusion of structure* in your eliciting and delivery of information. You should never just speak in a continuous flow, even if your thought processes are spontaneous and unstructured. You must give an illusion of structure. Do this by separating your thoughts into intelligent blocks, using pauses, and adding in some 'headings' and 'signposts'. Make it appear as though your thoughts are structured, and develop a way of speaking that sounds more structured than it actually is. A useful and powerful structuring tool is to mention that there are a 'number of (for example, treatment) options', and then separate out the options with 'firstly...', 'secondly...', and so on. Add in such structural components whenever you can. This is the scaffolding upon which you can construct your thoughts, and it makes your thought processes much more accessible and understandable to the examiner and patient/actor.

Establish the need

Finding out what the patient/actor actually needs from an interaction is often an important part of the key to unlocking the scenario. Your investigation will be much more effective if you understand the needs of the patient/actor. Sometimes in a scenario, a patient/actor will have *wants*, but these may be different to the *needs*. For example, they may *want* to have conservative medical treatment rather than elective surgery. Their want will be obvious. The *need* in the scenario is found by establishing the degree of surgical urgency. You can still usefully access the need by utilizing the want, even in this situation. You should never collude with a patient, but you must use what they offer you. Listen to what they want, and this will give you access to information regarding what they actually need—in this case, information that informs your view regarding urgency. So, the wants of a patient can be an access route into establishing their needs.

In scenarios where the objective is to explain something to a patient, you have to ascertain how much information the patient/actor wants and needs to know. This again is about establishing the need. If you are delivering bad news, you have to know the amount of detail that the patient/actor actually needs in this particular interaction. It may be too much to say everything now—and this is a good example of 'less is more'. You can indicate that there is more you could talk about, but perhaps they should make another appointment to do so. There are times when you *have* to deliver certain information, for example, when breaking bad news. It may be too much for them to hear that a partner has a diagnosis of cancer but, unfortunately, they will need to hear it. You must ensure that you deliver news like this very clearly and unambiguously. Be straightforward. Grasp the bull by the horns; don't beat around the bush (thereby illustrating my point with exactly what you should not do). (See the example in Box 12.2.)

BOX 12.2 GIVING WHAT IS NEEDED

For example, in a scenario where the candidate is asked to counsel the patient about a genetic disease, such as retinitis pigmentosa (RP), the approach must be tailored to the specific patient. RP has differing inheritance patterns. The advice given to a young woman planning a family, whose brother has x-linked RP, would be different to the advice needed by a man in his forties with two children who is losing his vision from autosomal recessive RP. Appropriate and considerate discussion is needed of the full family history, and the hopes and fears of the individual for their family, before giving bespoke advice, rather than just an all-out stock regurgitation of everything known about the inheritance patterns of genetic disease.

Being collaborative

A collaborative approach to health practice is a core tenet of a patient partnership model of health care, and is something we should all be aspiring to. It falls into our skills toolkit because a truly collaborative approach is a very powerful and effective way of both eliciting information quickly and of making the patient/actor (and examiner) recognize that you are being empathic and listening to their concerns. However, being truly collaborative can't be a passive skill we apply to every single OSCE scenario. That would be dangerous, since many of the scenarios require a more direct approach, particularly if the patient/actor is very unwell or vulnerable. Therefore, we must apply our skill of collaboration in a more calculated way.

You should never appear wholly paternalistic in the OSCE. As I mentioned previously, in some cultures, paternalism is an essential way of working since that is what the patient expects and needs. For the OSCE however, we must never be wholly paternalistic. Paternalism goes totally against the ethos of a patient partnership approach to care. On the whole, we should be working with the patient/actor, following clues that they give us, to find the key to the scenario. Remember, they have a script, so it is definitely in your best interest to work with them in revealing the content of that script. This is analogous to real life of course, when we are trying to investigate and follow a patient's real-life clinical narrative. Start from a position of total collaboration, and be less collaborative if that is required. Ask a patient/actor regularly if they understand what you are saying, and enquire if there is anything else you should know. Work with the patient/actor to solve the task—they are your collaborator in this OSCE.

Patient collaboration is essential for a fluid performance in physical examination stations. You need to give clear requests and instructions, and the patient/actor needs to cooperate with these. This is particularly important, for example, in a neurological examination when checking subjective sensation, and also when the instructions are precise and potentially confusing, such as during visual field testing.

Practise being collaborative in your study group, and build up a selection of tools that will help to encourage collaboration with your patient/actor. Build up a selection of phrases that make others want to collaborate with you. You can't force collaboration: the patient/actor must genuinely want to share and collaborate with you. You can only enable this by being empathic and saying the right things. They need to believe that you really care about what they think and feel. You can see, by now, how ineffective a paternalistic approach would be in this respect. Collaboration and effective empathy sit hand in hand, so use your empathy to access collaboration.

Taking charge

There are a few occasions during the OSCE when you will need to be firmer in your approach and take charge of an interview. However, these are very infrequent, and you should only take charge if you really need to. It is important always to control an interview to a certain extent, but you have to get the balance of being able to demonstrate an ability to control, with a wish to work collaboratively and be guided by the patient/actor. This is often a fine line.

Sometimes, you might need to take charge in a more subtle, covert way. For example, if the patient won't speak to you at all, you should be progressively gentler, whilst also being progressively more persuasive (as I previously described). However, there are also occasions when it is very important for you to demonstrate that you are taking charge in a very deliberate and obvious way. Indeed, it may be one of the things the examiner is looking for (see the examples in Boxes 12.3 and 12.4).

BOX 12.3 TAKING CHARGE

One occasion you may need to take charge is with a very talkative/manic patient, who simply will not stop speaking. These patients are very difficult to interview. To ask questions, you need to actually stop them speaking. You must do this by being more and more assertive and firm. A useful tactic is to combine some body language with your assertive statements. If you say 'please stop for a moment', and it doesn't work, try 'please stop', with a flat palm towards them. This hand gesture usually does the trick. Don't just speak over them.

BOX 12.4 DEALING WITH THREAT

Another occasion when it is essential that you actively and assertively take charge of the interview is when you feel threatened by a patient/actor. In this situation, it is worth telling the patient/actor that you feel threatened by them. If they continue, then you must say that if they do not stop you will terminate the interview. If they still continue, then stand up as though you are terminating the interview. Knowing when to leave a potentially dangerous situation is an important skill to possess, and an important one to demonstrate to the examiner.

Perhaps there are other situations you can think of, or have come across, where you overtly need to take control of an interview. However, please remember that this should only be done in exceptional circumstances. During a normal interaction, you will be in control, and you should demonstrate to the examiner that you are in control, but you should do so in a very subtle way that allows collaboration with the patient/actor. You need to perfect this fine balance.

Steering the ship

Candidates who are over familiar with the OSCE stations know exactly which way they will be steering their ship. They know the destination and are already aware of pitfalls on the way. They will have practised negotiating the pitfalls, and will be ready to get to their destination in the several minutes' long OSCE station. I realize that this approach provides a peace and security that many candidates desire, and that even reading this may give you some comfort. However, this is the wrong approach, and you risk failure in a scenario that has been subtly changed. A detective who assumed that every dead person found with a gun in their hand had committed suicide would be missing the clues that might otherwise steer them towards a more sinister case of murder.

You should not be entering any scenario with more than a rough idea of where you want to end up. Your final destination must be guided by your patient/actor and the form and content of the information you gather from them. They dictate the final destination, and, if you are a skilled investigator, you will let them dictate the route too, because a route dictated by a patient/actor will always be better than the pre-defined route with which you entered the scenario.

The skill in steering your ship is in knowing roughly where you want the interview to go and what information you need to elicit to make your way there, but being directed towards your actual route and final destination by any new information you receive. To be adept at this skill, you need to be flexible in your thinking, and you need cognitive room to manoeuvre in your approach. If you are too familiar with the route, you will find it very difficult to change direction during a stressful OSCE station.

Assessing impact

In any OSCE scenario, you should try to get a sense of how this person is affected by their illness, and what impact their illness has on their functioning and quality of life. This should always be in the back of your mind. This will help to inform your decisions regarding management, and may change your view on prognosis.

When you ask about symptoms, try to gain an understanding of how these symptoms impact on their day-to-day life. This is also useful because it will make you appear more empathic, and will give the patient/actor the impression that you really care about them (which you do, of course).

So, when asking about the character of the pain they experience at night, also ask how the pain affects them in other ways. For example, do they lose sleep? (See Box 12.5.)

BOX 12.5 EXPLORING THE IMPACT

For example, if a patient/actor has heart failure, how does that impact on their life? How does it affect them? Knowing this gives you access to lots of information, because you will be asking about the heart failure by asking about things that really matter to them. You will be addressing their actual concerns and anxieties, rather than just gathering information. So, ask how this affects them. Ask what their concerns are. Starting open, ask: how does this illness make them feel? How has it changed their life? Closing down, ask: how are they sleeping? How is this affecting their job? Indeed, are they working at all? How is this affecting their relationship?

When examining a patient, consider in what ways the physical findings might result in functional changes. Indeed, you may be expected to assess function formally in some physical examination stations (for example, in the assessment of rheumatoid hands).

Just add a flavour of impact investigation into aspects of your enquiry. With practice, you will learn how to do this quickly, and will also learn how much more efficient your investigation can be with a sense of the degree of impact. You need to integrate the impact investigation with the general enquiry. You can't effectively ask about characters of pain and then tag an impact enquiry onto the end. Seamless integration will give a more caring and empathic impression, and your further questions will be shaped by the degree of impact revealed.

Following a lead

If you take care to listen to everything a patient/actor has to say, and don't just concentrate on the responses and narrative that you feel are important at this moment, then you will occasionally capture pieces of information that you weren't expecting. These extra bits of narrative, sometimes provided spontaneously by the patient/actor, are potential *clues* in your investigation.

Once you've heard a potential clue in your OSCE scenario, you need to decide how much weight to assign to it. You should estimate how important it may or may not be to follow this lead. When you hear a potential clue in the OSCE, I would suggest that, as a minimum, you should verbally acknowledge the clue to the examiner. For example, if the patient/actor drops into the conversation that they have been feeling warm lately, say: 'You've been feeling warm? That's interesting', or something like that.

Once you have repeated the clue to emphasize it, you need to decide if this is a lead you want to follow and explore now. Be wary though, as you could be opening up a Pandora's box. For example, if you are assessing heart failure and the patient/actor says they have been drinking more alcohol recently, you need to acknowledge this new information, but then decide how far you want to pursue that line of investigation. It can take valuable time to complete a thorough alcohol history, and you might need to focus on the other cardiac risk factors in order to build up a more inclusive picture. Then again, it might be the case that alcohol is a crucial factor in this particular scenario, so adequately exploring this lead may be essential for success. You need to decide the weight of a potential clue at the time, and use your clinical judgement and acumen to inform your decision.

If you acknowledge a clue, and decide that it is important, but you don't have time to take it further, then say that to the patient/actor. Tell them that you would like to talk about it later, but now must, unfortunately, focus on the more pressing matters at hand. Be aware though that acknowl-edging the clue, and moving on in this way, is only done for the sake of the examiner. It is very unlikely that you will actually have time to cover this extra potential clue later in the scenario, and, unless you make a note of it, you will surely forget. I would recommend that if a clue presents itself that appears to justify further investigation, you should follow it there and then. Don't risk leaving it and forgetting about it. If you do want to leave it until the end, and you think it is important, try to make a quick written note of it (if notepads are allowed of course).

So, the best way to conduct an interview is to have a rough idea of where you are headed and to have the ability to steer the ship, but to be flexible and adjust course depending on whatever potential clues or icebergs the patient/actor leaves in your path. If you just plough straight ahead and ignore the icebergs, you may sink. Sometimes, the small clues that a patient/actor throws into a scenario are actually pointers towards the key that unlocks the scenario, and, sometimes, the key to a scenario is miles away from your original destination. So listen, and be guided by your patient/actor.

Body language

If you are anxious, your body language can give that away. Body language betrays the anxious candidate, so you shouldn't wear your heart on your sleeve in this examination. Learn to hold your posture and try not to fidget. Don't wring your fingers and don't play with your hair. Your body language should be exuding quiet, calm confidence no matter what you are actually feeling inside.

However, another more important reason to make your posture and body language one of *still calm* is that body language can be a powerful tool to employ in the OSCE. If you want to emphasize speech, a hand movement can be powerful, but only if that hand was previously still and calm. If you want to appear more caring when a patient tells you something very painful, you can subtly soften your posture—drop your shoulders slightly and lean into the patient very discretely, as though wanting to physically, as well as psychologically, contain their pain. Conversely, if a patient says something inappropriate or threatening, you can distance yourself by sitting up straighter and holding yourself firmer and more formally. In this very subtle way, you are communicating your objectivity and professionalism to them. However, any subtle body movement will only have power if your body was previously still and calm.

Always consider your body language during rehearsal, and use your posture for subtle, non-verbal communication. You should always be communicating quiet confidence to both the patient/actor and the examiner. Make sure that you aren't communicating anxiety. Your posture and body language is a subtle but powerful tool, the use of which you should practise in your study group. Use video recordings to examine your own body language, and modify your performance accordingly. Body language and non-verbal forms of communication are essential in the OSCE, and they should be rehearsed and perfected.

Active listening and vocal tics

Body language is one way that we can subtly communicate *active listening* to the patient/actor and examiner. Active listening makes the patient feel listened to and understood, encourages them to deliver more information, and reassures the examiner that you are actively engaged in the interac-tion. It gives the impression that you are interested. Practise your subtle head nods, eyebrow movements, smiles of encouragement, and empathic head shakes. If you need source material for this, then just watch any well-acted film.

When we actively listen to a patient/actor, we punctuate their speech by using verbal and non-verbal prompts that encourage them to elaborate further. The prompts represent our interest and understanding of what they are telling us, and should, in some way, distil and repackage the information we have just heard in a brief verbal or non-verbal way. During the OSCE, we are listening to every word, but whilst doing so, we are also operating on a much higher level: thinking about the overall direction of the interview; looking out for clues and red flags; subtly controlling the interview whilst working in collaboration with the patient/actor; being empathic; planning our strategy; and considering our next question. We therefore need to develop verbal and non-verbal prompts that can give the impression of active listening, without expending the time, energy, and focus required to do this for real.

To listen actively in the OSCE, we need to develop a collection of phrases to punctuate a patient/actor's narrative and encourage them to continue. The actual words are not as important as the way they are spoken, and it is crucial that the tone and intensity of the prompts are appropriate and in keeping with the current discourse. Such a collection might include: 'I see'; 'go on'; 'indeed'; 'I'm sorry'; 'really?'. The phrases should be generic, useable in most situations, and rotated as required.

However, be wary of vocal tics. You may find that, during a scenario, you tend to say a particular phrase time and time again. Often, this phrase can be inappropriate if you actually think about the words spoken, but you will continue to use it, as this is your solitary default phrase. A contender for this is 'okay'. A patient/actor may tell you something distressing that they think is certainly not okay, but you will not be thinking about the meaning of your vocal tic. Another type of tic is to just repeat the last couple of words of whatever the patient/actor has just said, although I know that some candidates find this very useful.

Develop a variety of short phrases that are comfortable for you, and practise using them to punctuate the patient/actor's narrative. Adjust the empathy tone so that the phrases sound empathically tuned to the tone and content of the patient/actor's speech. Become aware of prompts and vocal tics within your study group and help each other out. It is only possible to get this right with the help of an observer who can feed back any problems and progress.

CHAPTER 13

Build your skills toolkit, part 3: history taking

CONTENTS

Generic interview skills

We will now move on and start to build up some more specific history-taking skills that can be considered and selected for use if required. Whilst they are more specific, I have still tried to make my description of them as generic as possible, and some of these principles can be applied in many different scenarios. However, keep in mind the need to balance your focus on the task at hand with a more expansive approach. As a general rule, you should be focussed but always ready to take a step back and look at the situation more objectively. Be prepared to *cast a wider net* and then re-focus your interview, if needed.

Clinical narrative

As a health practitioner in training, we are taught ways to take a clinical history, conduct a clinical examination, or complete a practical procedure. It is important to start with a well-known pattern, plan, or structure. This is how methods are taught and passed down to a new generation of practitioners. In addition, the structure allows the senior colleague to understand where the junior practitioner is going. For example, the structured cardiac history, with cardiac risk factors listed after the history of the presenting complaint, tells the senior colleague what he needs to know and also directs the junior trainee to the salient historical factors. As a novice, we tend to use pre-set structures for our history taking in order to collect all of the necessary information required to formulate the case.

As we become more experienced, these learnt structures become second nature and we are more able to detect the subtleties of the interview process or practical procedure. It is much like a singer who knows how to read music, learns the piece, and then, once the mechanics of the delivery are second nature, is able to concentrate on the feel of the delivery. Singing the actual notes in the correct order is the bare essential: one must transcend that for a truly magnificent performance. As you become a master of history taking, the form of the history assessment changes, and you are more able to follow the *clinical narrative*.

When presented with a history-taking task in the OSCE, the examiner and patient/actor will have established a narrative for the candidate to discover. This clinical narrative is unique and specific for this particular history scenario, and the patient/actor will have a script that lists a narrative pattern for them to follow. In order for you to follow the clinical narrative of this particular scenario, you need to be confident and flexible, register every communication from the patient/actor (both verbal and non-verbal), and never embark on the journey sure of the final course or destination. Don't make assumptions based on similar scenarios you may have encountered. You should always cast a wider net and be open-minded. In this way, you use your skills to follow a collaboratively established clinical narrative, facilitated by your pertinent questions but, ultimately, guided and dictated by the patient/actor. You need to collect other historical points along the way, building up a bigger illness picture with ancillary facts, and checking for unusual 'red flag' features, facts, or symptoms. By the end of the assessment, you may have asked all the standard history questions, but using the clinical narrative to guide your direction, rather than a rote-learnt history structure, is more effective, thorough, and impressive.

Experienced clinicians usually have clinical narratives in mind, and this enables them to take fast, accurate, skilled histories from new patients. As an OSCE candidate, you need to write your clinical narrative from scratch, in collaboration with the patient/actor, and not just follow a narrative of illness that you may have come across before and suspect to be present here. Indeed, expert clinicians with a particular clinical narrative in mind may be at risk of making a mistake, perhaps missing something key that would change the final destination and formulation. Therefore, for true mastery, one should retain a healthy insecurity and inquisitiveness, and always write the collaborative clinical narrative from scratch.

Of course, OSCE candidates, approaching a familiar scenario, often fall into the trap of premature pattern recognition, and may plough along well-rehearsed and practised furrows, missing key facts along the way. Even a master can fall into the same trap. Always be wary of pattern recognition, even if that pattern is in the form of a sophisticated clinical narrative. Always be unsure inside, whilst appearing confident of course, and never commit to a final formulation of the case until you are at the end of the newly written clinical narrative.

So, try not to approach an OSCE station with a rote history in mind—be open-minded and write the clinical narrative in collaboration with the patient/actor. Indeed, your task in the OSCE station is not to recite a particular list of questions but, rather, to write the ideal questions for this particular scenario from scratch, in collaboration with the patient/actor. However, it is worth noting that how closely you 'stick to the script' of history taking depends on the level of examination the OSCE is part of. A first-year undergraduate student might be expected to just stick to the script, and candidates in an initial professional qualifying examination will not be expected to perform to the same standard as those in a specialist 'exit' OSCE examination. Be guided by your level of experience.

Assessing form, not content

This is an important concept when assessing health and illness—we have access to the *content* a patient gives us, but we are actually trying to assess the *form* of the illness. When we take a history, we ask questions to guide the patient's narrative structure, and we listen to their story. However, we must not get lost in the content. We must see beyond this to assess the form of an illness, using this to inform our diagnosis and treatment plan. Sometimes, the content gives us valuable information about the form, but we must only get a taste of the content. There simply isn't time, in an OSCE station lasting minutes, to indulge the patient/actor and listen to the content. We need to assess the form and move on.

Think of illness content as a murky and interesting pool of water. The patient/actor would love us to jump into the water and join them in the dark depths of intricate and often fascinating content. However, we must stand on the side of the pool and only dip our toes into the water. Once we have a feel of the temperature, we take our toes out and walk around to a different bit of the pool, and dip our toes in there. We just want a taste of the content to enlighten our understanding of the form.

You need to develop ways of politely moving the patient/actor on when they start telling you about the intricacies of their life. Do this in a caring and gentle way. However, you must move them onto the next bit of form you need to assess. You could say something like: 'That's interesting. Perhaps we could speak about that later?' It's probably better though to be a bit more honest and say: 'I'm sorry, I don't have time to talk about that right now. Could you tell me more about the chest pain?' At times, however, you may need to explore content a little more (see Box 13.1).

> ## BOX 13.1 EXPLORING CONTENT
>
> It is sometimes useful to get more specific knowledge regarding content. This is the case, for example, when assessing the possibility of biliary colic. In this situation, your access to the form is via specific content details, and you must lead the patient/actor along the pathway of their content-driven clinical narrative. It is important to know exactly what they are eating and how that is linked temporally to the abdominal pain. Here, the content enlightens our assessment of the form, but we are controlling the interview and only asking about as much content as we need.

Box 13.1 gives an example of when you need to subtly and covertly control the interview. You should never, ever, be sitting in the OSCE being bombarded with lots of content from the patient/actor. You only want as much content as you need to enlighten your assessment of form. So, practise subtle ways of controlling the content in order to access the form.

Assessing risk and urgency

Assessing risk and urgency is an important principle in health assessments and can be crucial in OSCE stations. No matter how straightforward things may appear on the surface, one must always be receptive to red flags and symptomatic markers of risk and urgency. We should always consider risk and urgency in real life, and I would suggest that this should never be far from your mind in the OSCE. To be receptive to factors that indicate risk and urgency, you need to listen carefully, have a good knowledge of features that could indicate something sinister, and be able to react accordingly.

Risk and urgency is critical in examinations and assessments of physical health, especially when going on to consider management plans in the OSCE. If you have examined a patient complaining of intermittent claudication, what are the other signs and symptoms present that may make this presentation more or less urgent? How would that change the information you deliver to the patient/actor in the scenario? Always try to consider how the degree of urgency impacts on prognosis and management, and incorporate this into your approach in the same way that you would in real life.

Consider capacity

Capacity is a key issue in every psychiatric assessment, but isn't just an issue for psychiatrists to deal with—whether or not a patient has capacity to consent to treatment is important for every health practitioner to consider. If you consent a patient for a procedure, do they have the sufficient capacity to sign the consent form? Capacity may not be explicitly tested in your OSCE (although it could be), but it is useful to consider capacity when you interact with a patient in any scenario, whether you are delivering or eliciting information, examining them, or performing a procedure. An understanding of capacity provides a useful way of structuring and formulating your view regarding the needs of the patient, in terms of what they can understand and what you should be telling them.

Remember that capacity is specific to a *particular* decision, for example, agreeing to a particular operation or treatment. A patient/actor may have sufficient capacity to make a decision regarding their choice of evening meal, but could possibly lack the capacity to make a decision about whether or not they should risk life-threatening surgery. Whenever you consider capacity, you are considering the capacity of a patient to make a *particular* decision—you should never form an opinion on the patient's overall capacity. A capacity assessment doesn't take long and it is usually worth having an idea about it, particularly if you are presenting results or discussing management with a patient/actor or consultant/examiner. Understanding capacity informs your management. So, if you ever need to present a management plan, always consider the patient's capacity to make decisions regarding your suggested management.

Capacity is established by a few simple considerations. Can the patient understand the information required to inform a particular decision? Can they retain this information for sufficient time to allow them to make the decision? Can they use the information in a balanced way to arrive at the decision? Finally, can they communicate their decision? (See Box 13.2.)

BOX 13.2 BEST INTEREST

If you come across an OSCE station where the patient's capacity is explicitly relevant (for example, the patient consenting to a life-threatening procedure), always remember that it is best practice for a patient/actor to be allowed to recover and regain their capacity to make a particular decision, in order for them to make that decision themselves. Always try to put the power of a decision into their hands. However, don't be scared to act in their best interest if the decision needs to be made immediately and they currently lack the capacity to make that decision. For example, a gastro-intestinal bleed might need an emergency investigation. If the investigation reveals that the treatment is non-urgent, the patient could be allowed to regain capacity before deciding whether or not to proceed with treatment. However, if the treatment needs to be done immediately, as an emergency, then you should act in their best interest and start it straightaway.

Capacity is a very important concept to master, and you need to consider the ethics surrounding your decisions regarding this. Going against a person's wishes, even if those wishes lead to certain death (for example, refusing a blood transfusion), is a very serious matter. When you present your decisions to an examiner, or a consultant in the linked scenario, be confident, but also be mindful that there is always a grey area when decisions concerning capacity are made. There is a fine line—you must not stand on the fence, but be aware that your opinion may not be shared by a colleague. Ethical considerations can also sway a decision of this nature. So, be confident in your view, but flexible in your stance: a rigid stance is easily broken.

Summarizing

Summarizing is a technique whereby you repeat back to the patient/actor pertinent features of your progress so far in the scenario. This is mainly to check with them that you have understood correctly, but can also fulfil the purpose of reminding the sleepy, non-attentive examiner what you have already covered. It can also allow you to structure and formulate your view and opinion, by effectively thinking aloud. I'm not a big fan of summarizing and I can't remember ever doing it, but it works well for some people. If you get stuck, it can be useful to go over things for the patient/actor, but I personally think, unless there is a specific reason for doing it, it serves little purpose.

However, if necessary, you do need to be able to summarize what you have learnt so far. This is particularly important in OSCEs with linked stations, when you may need to talk about the first scenario during the second linked station. To summarize a case in this way, it is important that you are very structured in your presentation. I would suggest that you practise presenting a normal structured history to someone else—get used to the flow. Then, you should structure your findings in this usual way, and present them in this standard format. Definitely don't try to present the information in the same way you elicited it. You need to restructure it and present it in a way that is easily understood.

Integrated history and examination

Integrating history taking with physical examination is a useful real-life skill, especially when time is short. It needs to be done carefully. We have considered the different approaches in terms of getting started and empathy tone in both history taking and examination, and, to integrate these, you need to balance your approach. Being too empathic during a physical examination may be inappropriate, since the patient/actor is partly undressed and the normal boundaries of personal space are breached by physical contact. Conversely, history should not be sought from the patient in a dispassionate way. So, to integrate these, you must tread a fine line in terms of your engagement with the patient/actor.

History taking should be guided by the clues present during the interaction, and these might include physical aspects of the patient/actor. For example, are they short of breath? Is there evidence of cigarette-stained fingers? Are they obese? Are there any visible scars? In this way, your history taking naturally integrates with observational aspects of the examination. This can be taken further, and it can be very powerful to guide your history by what you find on examination. However, to do so, you must rehearse effective and sensitive ways of combining questions with physical contact.

As a technique, it is useful to practise integrating history with examination, and indeed, you should not think of these things separately. They are both crucial elements of the basic information-gathering process that enables our formulation of the case and management plan. I will discuss physical examination in more depth in the next chapter.

Drugs and alcohol

Drugs and alcohol are not just the remit of the psychiatrist. There are many physical health conditions requiring medical and surgical intervention that are precipitated and perpetuated by drug and alcohol use. Enquiring about these can be like opening a Pandora's box, especially if you are in the middle of a complex history and you learn that the person has been drinking more alcohol recently. It can take a lot of precious time to get an accurate drug and alcohol history, and you need to decide how much weight to attach to this. You have to develop different depths of strategy, depending on how much time you have and, more importantly, how relevant the drugs and alcohol are to the matter at hand.

Screening the wider history

OSCE instructions are usually very specific. They will give you a precise task, and may even tell you bits of the history you *shouldn't* ask about. It would be very challenging to have to gather a full history in the fleeting minutes available to you, and, normally, your investigation will need to be more focussed. However, it is very useful to have the ability to sieve through the whole history and gain nuggets of information that will significantly inform your views on diagnosis, risk, urgency, and management.

You need to develop an efficient way of running through the full basic history structure in your head, and then dipping into this to pursue key points pertinent to the present scenario. In a patient with heart failure, you may focus more on cardiac risk factors; and in a depressed patient, you might be interested in wider social issues and past psychiatric history. It may be useful to consider and explore previous hospital contact, medication, and pre-existing physical health issues.

You should think of the history as a whole whenever you rehearse a scenario, making mental (not written) notes of the parts that might be useful. Then, practise running through these key points, in no more than a minute. If you do this during a modelling session, then the 'actor' will make up bits of information depending on the questions you ask and, therefore, your questions will be reinforced by adding to the narrative that you are creating as a group. If you ask relevant questions, then you will be forming a more complex and interesting scenario, and it will be more challenging for the next person to elicit that information.

During the actual OSCE, it is very useful to be able to quickly screen through the history and dip in for relevant questions. By developing this skill, you will be decreasing the chance of missing anything. Of course, a good assessment needs to be deep and focussed, and you can't always ask everything. However, by developing this screening and sieving tool, you can be systematic in your thinking, adding just pertinent and focussed questions that contribute to the depth of your overall interview. To do this, you must choose the questions carefully. So practise this important skill in your study group. This is also a useful skill if you freeze and get stuck—don't panic; just systematically pick out a couple of relevant screening points to get yourself moving again.

CHAPTER 14

Build your skills toolkit, part 4: practical skills

CONTENTS

Hands on

There are certain generic and psychological aspects to any physical examination or practical procedure, and we will consider a few of these here. If you can master your basic technique, contain any physical tells, and unravel any unhelpful psychological baggage, then you can concentrate fully on the challenging task at hand.

Physical examinations

In contrast to what I have previously advocated in this book, physical examinations should be learnt and rehearsed, like a dancer rehearses a routine. They should flow seamlessly and effortlessly, demonstrating to the examiner that you are not only skilled and practised in this examination, but that you can also spot any clinical signs, whilst making the patient feel contained at ease. The first time you are taught how to examine an abdomen, the teacher will impress upon you the importance of looking at the patient's face when you palpate. This is to ensure that you are not causing pain. This principle needs to be extended to any scenario where you are laying hands on a patient, or doing anything that could, in any way, cause harm or distress. You need to watch carefully for signs of discomfort or distress from the patient and react accordingly.

When conducting a physical examination, it is still important to maintain an appropriate *empathy tone*. This should be calming and containing, instilling the patient with confidence in your ability as well as your compassion. It should also be reactive to the patient—both in terms of what they may tell you during the examination, and how they may respond.

When perfecting your examination technique, consider ways you might combine aspects of your physical examinations in order to minimize the inconvenience to the patient. Divide the examinations up into body areas—for example, hands, arms, back, front—and group together the examination elements, irrespective of body systems. This can be useful if you need to perform an integrated examination, for example, a combined abdominal and cardiac examination. In real life, you will do this all the time: you will only examine a patient once, but you will examine all the body systems in that first, thorough screen. Perfect techniques of making this integration seamless, in a way that makes sense to the examiner.

It can be useful to *forward plan* whilst performing your physical examination. You may be expected to present examination findings to your examiner, and, if you can, forward plan your presentation and formulation while you work. For example, if you hear a murmur, then you can leave the stethoscope on the chest for a few more seconds, giving you time to consider the character of the murmur, and also time to structure your examination findings in your mind and to formulate a differential diagnosis.

Physical examination findings should be presented in a clear and structured way, demonstrating to the examiner that your thinking is methodical and clear. If you reach a definitive diagnosis, you need to explain why you believe that this is the diagnosis and how you ruled out the other possibilities. If you don't reach a definitive diagnosis, then presenting your findings in a structured way, followed by your list of differentials, may still gain sufficient marks. Don't rush straight into the key findings—be structured and methodical in your approach.

If you need to interact with the examiner, pitch your discussion or presentation at the level of someone in the next stage of your career. After all, the OSCE is the gateway to this next stage, and you are being tested for competency to move up to a higher level. For example, in a surgical fellowship OSCE, you need to discuss at the level of a new consultant. In a medical student OSCE, pitch your discussion at junior doctor level. Always maintain respect for the patient/actor, who will probably still be present, and speak to the examiner in the same way you would speak in front of a real-life patient. Continue to acknowledge the existence of the patient/actor—you are still in the simulation, and they are still a person who deserves consideration and respect. By speaking directly with the examiner, you are partly breaking the illusion of the simulation. However, you must maintain the reality of the presence of a patient/actor: never neglect or forget them.

Demonstrating practical skills

The OSCE is a test of clinical expertise, during which we need to demonstrate that, for us, the mechanics of the process are second nature, and that we are operating at a higher level where we can utilize this process to detect or treat pathology. However, we do need to strike a balance between what is expected from us at our level of training, and what our skills allow us to do. For example, as a trainee surgeon, you may have developed very personal and sophisticated ways of quickly completing a procedure successfully, with no complications. However, the examiner may want to see you do what they expect you to do—to follow the well-trodden path and not stray outside of that. In this case, it is not that the examiner wouldn't appreciate your skills or agree that your method wasn't good, but they may be concerned that you are running before you can walk. They may be tired and lacking concentration; they may be feeling anxious watching you do something they are not used to. Candidates may have trained in different institutions and countries where 'up-to-date' variations of techniques are in use. Not all examiners themselves will be familiar with, or even up to date with, all techniques. Therefore, if a standard way of approaching a practical skill exists, it is probably better to show that you are aware of, or have mastered this, before attempting any discussion or demonstration of more advanced techniques.

There are many reasons why an examiner could lose confidence in you when you don't follow the standard structure, and this is a risk that you shouldn't take. In the OSCE, you need to play it by the book, and stick to what is normal and expected. You want the examiner to feel comfortable and confident in your abilities, so they are likely to leave the scenario believing you to be a safe and competent practitioner. If you stray outside of an examiner's comfort zone, into new territories, he may feel anxious, even if what you are doing is good—and an examiner leaving a scenario feeling anxious about your performance is not a good thing.

Balancing empathy and pragmatism

When you are performing a procedure on a patient who is awake, you must be kind and compassionate, whilst also being totally in control in a containing, subtly paternalistic way. This is a fine balance. You can't just be empathic. You can't collaborate with them and connect emotionally—but you can understand that they are terrified, and you can offer some genuine words of care and comfort. The examiner needs to see this. You also need to demonstrate control and confidence, clinical precision and efficiency, and, actually, emotional distance from the patient.

Whilst it is possibly the case that the merging of technical and non-technical skills is the hallmark of surgical mastery, you need to be mindful of your level of training and abilities. I would suggest that you intersperse your clinical precision and emotional distance with moments of empathic checking that the patient is not in distress. Do this overtly, in the way you would show the driving instructor that you are now looking for traffic in the mirrors, but never lose focus of the main task in hand. The short bursts of caring and empathy will have greater impact because they are sandwiched between your overall clinical precision and excellence.

Containing procedural anxiety

The difficulty with procedural anxiety is that it is easier to spot objectively (for example, a hand tremor), it can actually impede your execution of the procedure, and it can make the examiner lose confidence in your procedural abilities. If your anxiety is obvious to you and the examiner, it can often be self-fuelling and perpetuating, and this is an extremely difficult cycle to break. It is probably the case that as soon as you pass your OSCE, the anxiety will dissipate, but, until then, you need to contain it at the very least.

Challenge negative cognitions

The key to containing procedural anxiety lies in understanding the cognitions that are fuelling this mental state. It is not possible to keep our physiology in check mentally, and we cannot will our hands to stop trembling, but we can develop mental techniques to get ourselves into a more positive frame of mind, to calm ourselves, and to settle our tonic resting state. The first step is to appreciate underlying negative cognitions and beliefs that are making our anxiety feel more unpleasant and distressing. We need to challenge those negative thoughts and beliefs, and realize that our trembling hands don't reinforce those beliefs. In fact, the trembling hands are just a normal physiological reaction. Separate out the physical manifestation from the underlying cognitions— sever those connections (see Chapter 4).

A cognitive safe place

The next step is to find a positive state of mind that enables and facilitates execution of the procedure in a calm and controlled way. This wouldn't necessarily involve thinking about anything specific, but it would be about creating a cognitive safe place into which you can escape and operate. The cliché is that of a safe cave, but the idea is that you create a safe place into which you can retreat while you clear your mind and focus on the task at hand. So, if you imagine your safe place, you need to visualize it and furnish it with items and details that you can easily remember. For example, it could be a book-lined library with an open fire and red velvet curtains, and you would have a nice comfy chair in front of the fire into which you sink at the start of the scenario. Outside the scenario, you should read the instructions, then take a few seconds to visualize your safe place. As you enter the scenario, imagine yourself entering the safe place and relaxing into a calm, composed state in which you can clear your mind and focus on the task at hand.

Breathing

Breathing technique is very important in scenarios involving demonstration of procedures. Anxiety can result in hyperventilation, and this can lead to tingly, clumsy fingers. Develop good breathing techniques, and ensure that your breaths are measured during your demonstration. Anxiety can lead to panic if a person hyperventilates—the build up of carbon dioxide sets up a positive feedback loop that makes the person feel more and more anxious. Stay in control of your breathing.

Rehearse

Rehearsal is key to containing procedural anxiety, and you should rehearse your technique, within timed examination conditions and under the watchful eye of a senior colleague, whenever possible. It may be useful to rehearse, mentally, the steps you'd take before a procedure in real life. For example, visualize scrubbing and donning surgical gloves before suturing. Familiarize yourself with the practical procedure, and build up a strong procedural memory pathway. This will allow you to fall back into a comfortable, second-nature technique when you perform in the OSCE.

Simulated composure and urgency

The OSCE is a simulation of real life, and we must play our role in this simulation. Just as we should be projecting empathic warmth when collaborating with a patient/actor to elicit or deliver information, we must also project the appropriate composure and urgency when demonstrating certain practical procedures. Just as our empathy must be turned up in this artificial simulation of life, so must our composure and urgency during simulated procedures.

When demonstrating a practical skill, we will be feeling anxious about doing so correctly, and we will be carrying the weight of the OSCE on our shoulders. As such, we cannot possibly naturally inject the required composure or urgency that would be appropriate in the real-life scenario, so we must do so purposively. We must play our role by simulating, albeit subtly, the appropriate tonic state for a given scenario, as though we were acting in a medical drama for television.

As with all OSCE stations, take this scenario very seriously, and respect the real-life simulation. You are demonstrating your global understanding of this procedure to the examiner, and this includes the tonic state you would be in if it were a real-life situation. Simulating composure is something that needs to be done throughout the OSCE, and this includes hiding physical tells and speaking in a calm and measured way. You should not be rushed; you should breathe carefully; and, recognizing that adrenaline is making you operate faster, you should be forcing yourself to slow down slightly.

There are certain procedures that may be time-limited in real life, and where technical speed and agility is important. In these scenarios, you should not rush, but you should operate quickly, as you would in real life. This might include a very slick technique for gripping a suture or using a piece of equipment. Be sure to go slow at crucial points, and then fast when you can, to simulate urgency and to communicate your understanding of the need for urgency.

With practical procedures, it is crucial that you treat the OSCE stations with respect and take the simulation very seriously. It is also important that you develop an understanding of underlying cognitions that fuel your feelings, and think about how you need to adapt your execution of the procedure to be true to the real-life equivalent.

CHAPTER 15

Build your skills toolkit, part 5: challenging scenarios

Dealing with challenging scenarios

Here are a few examples of different challenging scenarios you may come across, and some suggestions as to how you might deal with them. You need to develop robust strategies that can carry you through every potential scenario you encounter. Whilst your approach will need to be formulated during the actual scenario, depending on how the patient/actor presents on the day, you can develop some generic skills to deal with them. Remember that when a patient/actor really starts 'acting', it is very difficult to deal with, in an already challenging situation. You need to deal with their 'acting' in an effective way, and pull them back to their script as quickly as possible.

The crying patient

I touched on this before—it is very tricky and needs to be handled very gently. If a patient/actor starts crying, you must stop speaking. Pause. Give them a bit of space. Then make a short, empathic statement such as: 'I'm so sorry.' Pause again. Then ask them, gently, if you can continue with the interview. Do not speak over them. Do not offer them an imaginary tissue. A good actor takes their craft very seriously, and if they are able to generate real tears, then they have probably accessed that emotion by thinking about something very real and emotive to them. (You, of course, have done the same thing, to add weight to your empathy.) So, you must treat a crying patient/actor with extreme caution, and be very gentle in your approach.

The paranoid patient

If a patient/actor is very paranoid and unwilling to speak to you, try to normalize the encounter, and take it away from them being 'mad' or even 'unwell'. Tell them this is routine, and the questions you are asking are unusual but you ask everyone the same questions. You are looking for form, but you may need to listen to, and even collude with, the content they tell you. However, do this very carefully, and only enough to get the information flowing. If they say: 'They are watching me!', you can collude with that statement by saying: 'Really? That must be terrible.' You are being honest—for them that must seem terrible. With a paranoid patient/actor, you need to get your hands dirty and enter into their world in order for them to open up. You can't just be dispassionate and say: 'Hmm, that's interesting.'

Patients/actors can be paranoid in all types of OSCE, and it is important to try to establish the source of their paranoia. Assuming that this is not a psychotic process, the paranoia is usually driven by fear and anxiety, uncertainty, and perhaps a lack of confidence in your abilities. It is worthwhile trying to establish the root cause of the paranoia and, at the very least, spending a few moments to reassure the patient/actor that they are in safe hands.

If a patient/actor is paranoid, don't just ignore this and plough onwards. This needs to be acknowledged and dealt with. The paranoia will either be a planned component of the OSCE scenario, or, if not, will be very alarming for the examiner to witness. If a patient/actor is genuinely paranoid, then that is as important as if they were in pain during a physical examination. The paranoia needs to be acknowledged and your approach modified accordingly. Perhaps you have been too brisk and insensitive? Perhaps you have said something that worried them? Try to get to the bottom of the paranoia.

The guarded patient

If the patient/actor is guarded, you need to be very gentle and try to gain access to them from different angles. The more you try, and the more frustrated you feel, the ever more gentle you need to be. Try to work out why they are so guarded. This will inform your way forward. If they are paranoid, then see the previous section. Often, the guarded patient/actor is fearful of something, but perhaps there is a more sinister reason why they are guarded? As previously mentioned, you may need to collude initially to get them to open up. Try to engender their trust in you as a practitioner and as a person. We are all human, and overtly trying to understand this difficult situation from their perspective will help them to open up.

The angry patient

Dealing with an angry patient/actor is a core skill, essential for all of us. How you deal with them depends on why they are angry. So, you need to understand their anger. Such understanding will show you the way forwards, and the way forwards depends very specifically on the particular context of their anger. However, you need to be in control of the interview, whilst still being gentle and understanding. Don't let the patient/actor control you. If you feel threatened, then you must tell them that their behaviour is inappropriate and that you feel threatened. If they continue, tell them that you will terminate the interview. In real life, the threshold for actually terminating an interview should be a lot lower than the threshold in the OSCE. However, you should still say that you will terminate the interview if you really feel threatened.

To defuse anger, you need to understand the source, so it is essential that you uncover the real needs and concerns of this patient/actor. The more you tell a person not to be angry, the angrier they will become. Anger must be understood and sympathized with, whilst maintaining control and boundaries. If a patient/actor shouts, then you must try not to react to this. You should contain them with calming words and physical body language. You need to de-escalate the situation, and this is done by demonstrating your understanding, by empathizing, by reasoning, and by giving a clear explanation of your concerns and motives.

The angry relative

The previous section is relevant to this one, and, if you feel threatened, you should inform the relative and say you will terminate the interview. You need to understand their anger, and should ask them to help you with this. It is usually obvious why a relative is angry, and you may not be able to defuse their anger: they are often angry because of what you are telling them. It is a difficult but necessary part of health care to tell relatives (and patients) things they do not want to hear. If you are telling a husband that his wife needs to be admitted to hospital, he may become angry. He may agree that she is unwell, but his initial response might still be one of anger. When you are saying something to a relative that makes them angry, you must be confident and firm in your opinion. You should be very sure that this is the correct decision. You need to be more containing and paternalistic than you would be with a patient. An angry relative expects and needs paternalism from you, and only with confidence and paternalism can you defuse their anger or, at least, help contain it. With their emotions contained, you should then tell them that you understand that this is very difficult, but that you will see them again to discuss it further if they wish.

Often, anger in a relative will stem from anxiety. You need to identify this anxiety and contain it. An angry mother is surely an anxious and worried mother. You need to recognize this and address the core concerns directly, making sure you don't give false hope and unrealistic reassurances. Be matter of fact, but very gentle. Be confident and subtly paternalistic since they need to really trust that you are a professional and an expert, and that their child is safe in your hands.

The sad patient

Be very gentle, and be guided in the manner of your approach by their presentation. Try to make the history questions follow their responses in a way that tells their story. You need to strike the balance of seeing the world through their eyes, but not being too patronizing or condescending—you can't possibly understand their pain, and it may offend them if you suggest you can. However, you can try to see their situation from their perspective, and if you do so, they will respect you for it. You may need to collude with their negative, distorted view of life in order to gain their trust and access their inner thoughts and feelings. By this I mean, for example, that you should agree that a particular thing sounds terrible and distressing. Attempt to understand their pain and let them know you are trying to see the world through their eyes, whilst reasserting the fact that you can't possibly really understand their pain—this is a fine and difficult balance.

The talkative patient

This can be very challenging, especially if the patient/actor is very good and passionate about being talkative and pressured in their speech. The most extreme version of this is a manic patient/actor, and, in such a scenario, it can be almost impossible to stop them speaking, let alone conduct an interview. You need to try to take control of the interview. Firm commands, combined with a firm hand movement, might be enough to stop them briefly, but they will soon set off again and you must think fast and ask questions fast. You need to follow their speech, and dip in with a question that has some relevance to what they are actually saying. It is no good trying to shout questions over them, but, for example, if they are talking about their social life in detail, you could ask if they have been feeling more confident lately. Often the type of questions you would like to ask a manic patient/actor, in order to investigate the depth of their pathology, will pique their curiosity and pander to their grandiosity. So, use this to your advantage.

Turned down, a talkative patient/actor can be difficult to interview, even if they are not overtly manic, and it is necessary to take control of the interview in a compassionate way. This is a balancing act, since you must take into account other aspects of the interview we have previously discussed: understanding the *wants* of a patient/actor to access their *needs*, and hearing the *content* of their delivery to access the *form* of their illness. With these factors in mind, and with a subtly controlling approach, a talkative patient/actor can be extremely useful.

The chaotic patient

It can be very difficult to make sense of a chaotic patient/actor, and extremely challenging to pull their rambling narrative into a structure that is easy to follow and investigate. Investigate the form of their illness, rather than the specific content. You may need to collude with them in order for them to open up, and to follow the twists and turns of their chaotic narrative. However, do so cautiously. If the patient/actor is disordered in their narrative structure, then you need to be very structured in your approach and questions. In this case, you are not fully guided by their answers, since you must retain a very systematic and logical approach to your questions. However, the final destination is still, ultimately, guided by their responses. You just need to apply a greater degree of structure in your investigation of their clinical narrative. Remember to dip your toes into the water to get a taste of the illness content, but then move onto the next parts of your investigation, to dip your toes into other areas. The content only enlightens your understanding of the form. You need to try to make sense of their rambling content and formulate it into something that is understandable, diagnosable, and, eventually, treatable.

The weary consultant

Some OSCEs require you to roleplay a discussion about a patient/actor with a senior colleague. When presenting to a consultant, you need to be very clear and very structured in your approach. Always assume that they are weary and barely listening. You need to give short, simple sentences. Start with a statement that summarizes how serious you think the situation is, and, in a sentence, give the outcome. For example: 'I would like to speak to you about this man I have just assessed. I am very concerned about him and I think he is unsafe to be discharged.'

Then, you need to say you are going to present the history. Don't just speak—tell the consultant what you are going to present. Highlight important positives and negatives. Present the case in the standard format, not in the order you elicited the information. Don't be patronizing, but check that they understand you. Be respectful of their authority and superior knowledge, but remember that you are a colleague.

Be confident, but not too confident. Give a firm opinion; do not sit on the fence. Be flexible, and be open to advice and suggestions if they don't agree with your management plan. Strike the balance of being confident in your opinion, but respectful of theirs. Be objective and dispassionate, but inject passion if you need to emphasize seriousness or urgency. Passion can be powerful, but use it very cautiously and in small doses.

The junior multi-disciplinary team member

Whenever you are speaking to another member of the multi-disciplinary team, whatever their level of experience, you are speaking to a colleague. Their opinion is as important as yours, and you must take care not to patronize them. However, they may be looking to you for guidance, so give guidance when they want it. Assess their need, and fulfil that need. Be confident, but not cocky. Ask them what they think. Collaborate with them, particularly in the formulation of a management plan. Speak to them like a colleague, not a child—but don't use jargon. Be clear and structured, and demonstrate leadership.

CHAPTER 16

Generic strategies

CONTENTS

Outline for a generic plan

A generic strategy for the OSCE is not a magical blueprint that gives all the answers to any station. It is actually a simple and logical structure that can provide a scaffold onto which the work carried out with tools from the skills toolkit can be applied. The OSCE scenario needs to be solved by hard work, using the skills you carry with you, and can't be solved by knowing the exact blueprint and route before you even walk into the station. The strategy you have in your mind beforehand needs to be simple and easy to work with. It needs to be malleable and easily influenced by the patient/actor and the obstacles they throw into your path. A rigid strategy is easily shattered and broken; a malleable strategy is actually stronger.

I suggest that a generic strategy for an OSCE scenario should have no more than five bullet points, and should be along the lines of the structure in Box 16.1.

BOX 16.1 A GENERIC STRATEGY

1. Focal problem
2. Casting a wider net
3. Moving forwards
4. Forming an opinion
5. Getting everyone on board

---

1. Focal problem

Almost every OSCE station will have a focal problem which needs to be searched for from the outset, and, in some cases, tackled first. The focal problem is not necessarily representative of the OSCE *construct*, but will be linked to this underlying construct in some way (see Box 16.2).

> ## BOX 16.2 **FOCAL PROBLEMS**
>
> - In a scenario where you are assessing the cardiac risk factors in a man who has had an infarction, the focal problem is the infarction itself, the initial event.
> - In a scenario where you need to decide whether or not blindness is hysterical, the blindness is the focal problem.
> - In a physical examination scenario, the focal problem may only become obvious when you have examined the patient/actor and discovered some abnormal findings.

Unlocking the focal problem

In the first situation in Box 16.2, you can tackle the focal problem directly, and ask details about the initial event, for example: 'Where was the pain?'; 'When did it start?'; 'Has this happened before?'; 'How were you found?'. In the second situation, the focal problem is a bit more tricky and needs to be tackled gently by gaining trust and acquiring information regarding the blindness, combined with a physical examination. However, unlocking the focal problem is still the primary objective and first part of our generic strategy, even if more work has to be done before it can be unlocked. In the third situation, the patient/actor may sometimes be wholly unaware of the underlying focal problem. Sometimes, the focal problem is to find out what the parent actually *needs* from you (see Box 16.3).

> ## BOX 16.3 **ESTABLISH THE NEED**
>
> You may be in a scenario where a concerned parent wants to ask you about their child's recent diagnosis of leukaemia. In this case, the focal problem is to find out what the parent actually needs from you, as the whole point of this scenario is to address these needs adequately. If you are in any explaining-type scenario, the focal problem is to establish the need and decide at what level you will pitch the information. How much do they want to know? How much do they already know? A scenario like this is not about your knowledge of childhood leukaemia but, rather, about what the relative wants and needs from you at that particular time.

Exploring the focal problem

You need to explore the focal problem in a robust and thorough way. In the example of the person who has had an infarction, you need to really investigate the facts and history surrounding the infarction. Of course, by doing this, you are actually making an assessment of the seriousness of the event. So, in fact, assessing the seriousness is the focal problem. I hope you can see, in this example, that even if you don't realize that the initial objective is to assess the seriousness of the event, by thoroughly exploring the focal problem, you will still be doing the same thing. Furthermore, as far as the examiner is concerned, you are actually assessing seriousness.

When you are in a scenario dealing with a parent, the first thing you should do is find out what they need from you. What are their concerns and anxieties? Once you know this, you can be sure that you are telling them what they need to know, rather than just speaking about an illness. It is *their* child who is ill, and you should be collaborative in your approach to discussing that with them. Constantly check that you are addressing their needs, and are speaking with the appropriate depth—not too much and not too little.

Rethinking the focal problem

I suggest that until you really understand the focal problem, you can't move forwards at all. If you think you have understood it, and then the patient/actor continues to be very difficult and distressed at a later point in your assessment (even at stages four or five of your generic strategy), you need to go back to stage one and rethink the focal problem. It is never too late to do this. You may need to jump back to stage one and make a course adjustment to your direction of travel. Bear in mind that you can pass an OSCE station in the last few moments, so never, ever, think it is too late to save it. However, you must be sure that you have established the right focal problem because, without this, you cannot possibly pass the station.

If the focal problem is trickier to get to, you need to find a gentle way in. Even if this seems impossible, and you are panicking on the inside, you must remain calm and gentle on the outside. You should be relentlessly calm, and then walk carefully forwards through the clinical narrative, collecting a flavour of the illness content to enlighten your understanding of the illness form.

Sometimes, it might be the case that the focal problem isn't what you initially thought it was, or what you expected it to be. You may think you understand the nature of the focal problem, and so you start on your journey. You circle the pool of illness content, dipping your toes into the water to get a flavour of the content in order to enlighten your understanding of the form. If there is chaos, then you will be very structured in your approach. However, the actual focal problem may be something completely different, and you may only be able to identify it by moving onto step two of your generic strategy: *casting a wider net*.

2. Casting a wider net

Once you have made a thorough investigation of the crime scene and collected all the possible clues pertaining to the focal problem, you need to take a step back and cast a wider net. This isn't just about asking wider questions concerning the focal problem itself, though it may include that. It is actually about taking a step back and thinking outside of the box, and then approaching the focal problem from a different perspective. This is important to make sure you haven't missed or misunderstood something vital. There may be some other aspect to the focal problem that you haven't yet considered. By taking a step back, we can ensure we cover all the bases (see Box 16.4).

BOX 16.4 STEPPING BACK

If you are a detective, and have thoroughly investigated the scene of the crime, you would then take a step back and think about the crime scene objectively and through different eyes. By doing this, you may notice that the door to the study was locked from the inside. So how did the murderer get into the room? Then you might realize that something is missing and a key fact that might help explain this discrepancy is absent. So, you check the windows and notice that one of them has been tampered with so that it could never be locked. This tampering probably happened before the crime itself, and had to have occurred from the inside of the house. In this way, you narrow your suspects down to people who had access to the house.

This is the essence of casting a wider net. In the example of our patient/actor who suffered an infarction, you cast a wider net by asking about the period of time leading up to the event. Was he stressed? What was his social and financial situation? What had changed in his life recently? Did he have previous angina symptoms? Is there any other evidence of critical ischaemia, such as limb claudication? Does he have previous history of this? Any previous medication, or contact with services? This is a relatively straightforward example of casting a wider net, and, to do it, you will be employing several skills from your toolkit. You will be sieving through his full history, very quickly, in order to gather nuggets of information that inform your wider understanding of his current situation.

In the example of explaining leukaemia to a concerned relative, you have already established the focal problem. You have a good idea what they need from you in this interaction. You can cast a wider net in this situation by asking questions surrounding the child's illness. Although this is an explaining scenario, there may be some important facts you need to guide your progress in this situation. Are they afraid of bereavement? Are there more immediate concerns, such as the need for chemotherapy or blood transfusions? You cast a wider net to gain an understanding of how the leukaemia impacts on the child's and family's lives. Once you have gathered all the information, you can move forwards in the right direction.

In the example of hysterical blindness, you have integrated your history and examination and have a good idea what the focal problem is. You cast a wider net by investigating what was going on in her life before the blindness, and what led to this event. With the physical examination example, you consider other investigative components that may add to your understanding of the clinical picture. For example, you may wish to add some neurological components into an eye examination scenario that appears to be indicating an underlying diagnosis of multiple sclerosis.

By thoroughly assessing the focal problem, then stepping back and casting a wider net, you are now in possession of a compass setting for this journey, and you know which direction you need to travel in. You don't yet know your final destination, but you know which direction you are travelling in. Knowing the direction allows you to move onto step three of the generic strategy: *moving forwards*. You can't move forwards until you know the compass setting.

3. Moving forwards

You have established the nature of the focal problem and have cast a wider net—now you move forwards in the direction that the first two stages of your strategy have allowed you to calculate. Moving forwards involves using your content and process skills, and working though the main objectives of the scenario.

Moving forwards may involve: further assessing of risk factors in the man who has suffered an infarction; explaining leukaemia, chemotherapy, and its side-effects to concerned parents; a thorough eye assessment to rule out physical causes of visual loss in a case of hysterical blindness; or a neurological examination in a patient you suspect may have multiple sclerosis. Move forwards in a particular direction, towards a final destination, using the generic skills you have in your 'back pocket' to engage, to elicit or extract information, and to negotiate any pitfalls you may encounter on the way.

Establishing direction

If a candidate is very familiar with a particular scenario, then they will try to move forwards through the task straightaway. Some candidates seem to think that this is how you pass the OSCE—it isn't. You can't just walk into a station and start moving forwards, since you first have to be sure that you are moving in the right direction. You have to set the scene and get the patient/actor on the same page: let them know that you are there to address their needs and concerns. You have to cast a wider net and check whether there is anything else factual that may change your course setting. After all this, you can then start to move forwards.

You can't move forwards along a pre-set route, and you can't know how you will actually move forwards until you are in the scenario itself. You will feel as though you need a particular route to follow, and this is why candidates are so keen to memorize OSCE scenarios. However, this does not necessarily lead to success in the OSCE. The route can't be predetermined; it must be worked out during the scenario. All you can do is have a very comprehensive and powerful skills toolkit ready for use, and move forwards in the best way you can.

Whilst moving forwards in the OSCE scenario, you need to have a low threshold for casting a wider net as you progress. This might be in the form of taking a step back and sieving through the wider history points. You should always be ready to step back and think more objectively about the task, otherwise you may miss something. For example, if the patient/actor drops in a statement about things being financially difficult, and you realize you haven't asked about their employment situation, take a step back and ask the relevant questions and any others that might be important. In this case, as well as establishing their employment history, it might also be important to have an idea about their level of education, or to know if they have outstanding debts. Always be ready to cast a wider net.

Striking a balance

Whilst moving forwards, you need to be there, in the scenario, with the patient/actor, focussed on them and on the task at hand, and reacting to the subtleties in their presentation. You need to be totally 'in the moment'. However, you also need to be able to step back, think, and be objective. This is a fine balance, but being able to balance apparently conflicting approaches and ideas is how you will be successful in the OSCE. Success is often about balance. The patient has to feel that you are being collaborative, and you need to be guided in your investigation by them, but at the same time, you need to be covertly (or sometimes overtly) in control of the interview. This is a balance. If you can be in the moment, whilst also watching from afar, you will make your performance in the task more bulletproof.

Moving forwards through the task allows you to gather the information needed for stage four of your generic strategy: *forming an opinion*.

4. Forming an opinion

By forming your opinion in the OSCE scenario, you are getting off at the last stop, at your final destination. You hope that, after all your work, you have reached the correct final destination. You don't need to fully commit yourself right away. There is still time to think and cast around for more guidance. For example, this might be a good time to ask the patient/actor/parent if there is anything else important you should know.

Remember that it is never too late to change your final destination in the OSCE, and success in a scenario can happen in the last few moments. It may be in the last minute, having explored the cardiac risk factors in detail (as you were asked to), when you ask him if there is anything else you should know, he mentions perhaps something about his personal life. Following the lead, you discover that he has recently started taking sildenafil. You are now in the last 40 seconds, but you can quickly establish the chronological link between this new crucial piece of information and his presentation. Establish this antecedent factor before the final bell rings, and you just might pass the scenario.

So, never be scared to take a step back and think outside of the box; never be cautious in casting a wider net; and allow yourself the space to change your final destination and re-form your opinion, even in the last minute of the task.

Collaboration

When you form your opinion, it is better to do this in collaboration with the patient/actor, and allow them to modify and guide your opinion, if necessary. However, this should be balanced by your confidence that your opinion is correct. You need to sound and act confident, but to allow yourself enough space and caution to change your opinion. Don't commit to a final opinion before you need to. Remain as flexible and as malleable as you can before finally being confident about what you think.

The same goes for an explaining scenario or a physical examination. Don't feel as though you have finished until you have cast a wider net and collaborated with the patient/actor/parent in the last few moments of your journey towards the final destination. Is there anything else they need to know or that you need to do? Have you adequately and properly fulfilled the requirements of this task?

Remaining open-minded

It is more straightforward to think of stage four of your generic strategy when considering the first example, that of the man who has had an infarct. You need to form an opinion, but, even though you may have had a good idea about this from the start, you should be open in your opinion until the very last moment. This is important on many levels. The patient/actor and examiner need to feel that you are open and investigating with no prejudice, otherwise you may find progress and information gathering rather tricky from a defensive patient/actor. You can only make an important decision if you have made a thorough and non-prejudiced open assessment. Also, suppose you had learnt, early on in the scenario, that this patient was a heavy smoker? You might have assumed this to be the main contributing cardiac risk factor, and could possibly have missed the critical change in medication that turned out to be your key to success.

Having formed your opinion, be confident and be sure that it is the right one. Once you feel that you are at your final destination, you can move onto the last stage of your generic strategy: *getting everyone on board.*

5. Getting everyone on board

This is a very important part of any OSCE scenario, and, if the earlier parts of the task have gone well, then it should be quite straightforward. However, trying to get everyone on board might result in a distressed and angry patient/actor who doesn't think he needs to be admitted, or distressed parents who are unhappy with even the fact that their child has been diagnosed with a serious illness. These reactions to your perhaps perfectly correct strategies and opinions will probably be part of the scenario, and delivering difficult and sometimes unwanted information is a very challenging part of our job as health practitioners (see Box 16.5).

BOX 16.5 CONTAINING ANXIETY

Once you have discussed leukaemia with the concerned parents, you may find that they are very distressed and overwhelmed by what you have said. You need to try to get them on board by containing their anxiety and reassuring them, if possible. When you leave the encounter, they should be feeling reassured and not too distressed. It may be that you tell them that this has been very difficult, and perhaps they should come and see you again to discuss it further. Perhaps give them some information leaflets to take away. Perhaps apologize if you have told them too much (though this is merely a courtesy, because you will have been constantly checking the appropriate level of information delivery). Strike the balance of being gentle and containing, but also being objective and not giving false hopes or reassurances. You understand how difficult this is for them, and their distress is to be expected. You must work hard to try and contain their stress.

Sometimes getting everyone on board is simply a matter of checking with the patient/actor that they are satisfied with the encounter. Sometimes it may be more challenging to get everyone on board. The man with cardiac risk factors may be unwilling to accept that his new-found passion needs to be sacrificed for the sake of his health. The patient with what you consider to be hysterical blindness may be very unhappy with your conclusion. In the case of a physical examination, you may need to get the examiner on board by presenting your findings, diagnosis, and management plan.

Of course, all is not lost if the final bell rings before you manage to get everyone on board with your opinion. The essence of the task can be completed the moment you get off at the last stop of your journey, and, sometimes, a scenario can be passed even if you don't reach the final destination. If you have been travelling in the right direction, and have asked the right questions, and thought about the scenario in the right way, you may pass anyway. Remember that it is much better to be halfway up a ladder that is facing in the right direction, than at the top of a ladder that is pointing the wrong way.

Resolution

Getting everyone on board gives you a sense of resolution and completion to the scenario. This may not be critical for the outcome, but can have a significant impact on your own mental state as you move onto the next OSCE station in the circuit. Being able to shake off feelings of frustration and disappointment from a previous scenario is critical in performing optimally in future ones, and resolving your scenario is a way to help this process. However, the best way to shake off a disappointing performance is to focus entirely on this new scenario, and don't allow yourself to dwell on anything that has occurred previously.

Afterword

CONTENTS

Taking control

The OSCE is a highly charged emotional experience, and it becomes more emotionally intense with subsequent attempts. In this book, I have tried to help you find ways to consider your emotions from a more objective standpoint, and we have spent time dissecting our thoughts, feelings, and beliefs from the cognitive processes surrounding our OSCE study and execution. I have encouraged you to think actively about emotions and feelings in the context of your clinical skills, and a colleague said to me, in my final stages of writing this book, that perhaps encouraging trainees to be *more* emotional during the already emotional OSCE might not be a good idea. In reply, I pointed out that the OSCE is emotional anyway, and by explicitly considering our emotions objectively, we are better equipped to package them up and segregate them. By being a bit more analytical of the cognitive processes at play during the OSCE, we are more able to be a master of our emotions, rather than being a slave to them.

Unhelpful truths

I am writing this book in the two years following illness and a neurosurgical operation, and the narrative, in some ways, mirrors my own recovery. This has been a very difficult time in my life, and whilst my operation was a 'success', I remained a 'failure'; although I was 'fixed', I somehow remained 'broken'. During my recovery, I lost someone. I felt alone and abandoned, and believed that this was why I remained broken. This was possibly partly true, but it was an unhelpful truth. As long as I held onto the belief that I was broken because I'd been abandoned, I was also stuck since I therefore needed a reconnection in order to heal. While I focussed on this, I was not allowing myself to deal with the other underlying issues that also caused me pain—the post-traumatic stress of the illness and operation itself.

A belief that resolves the conflict of 'success' and 'failure', even if there is some truth to that belief, is unhelpful. It diverts your attention and stops you from dealing with other important underlying issues. It may be true that the OSCE is in some ways flawed, but this is a distracting truth that is unhelpful to you and puts you at a disadvantage to first-time candidates. I can't reconnect, and you can't change the OSCE. Only by shedding these distracting superficial beliefs can we deal with the real underlying issues that are causing us pain in life.

Embrace the positive

If you are unlucky enough to fail the OSCE, or perhaps have already failed when you read this book, then you need to make every effort to use your previous experience in a positive way, and try not to dwell on the negative. This may be extremely difficult, particularly if you have already failed more than once. However, remember that having already attempted the examination, you are actually at an advantage to first-timers, since you know exactly what to expect and will be less distracted by the setting and experience as a whole.

Change

If you have failed a few times and are feeling disheartened, do not give up—try again. However this time, change your entire approach. Change your attitude to the OSCE and to your College. Change your approach to study and rehearsal. Break the exam down, and don't let it break you. After failure, you definitely should not be using the same old technique to study: modify your approach. Please do not simply indulge your anxiety by immersing yourself, once again, in the content and by re-learning the scenarios. This will merely fuel your anxiety.

At the very least, I hope this book has made you think about the OSCE in a slightly different way. It is useful to approach any tricky obstacle in your life from different angles, especially if you are initially unsuccessful. Try to lose any baggage, and develop your skills from the ground up, constructing your strengths as you deconstruct the task at hand. Break everything down into its component parts, and from that, you will build an arsenal of generic skills and strategies that will allow you to sail through any scenario you encounter.

Good luck!

Appendix: Workbook

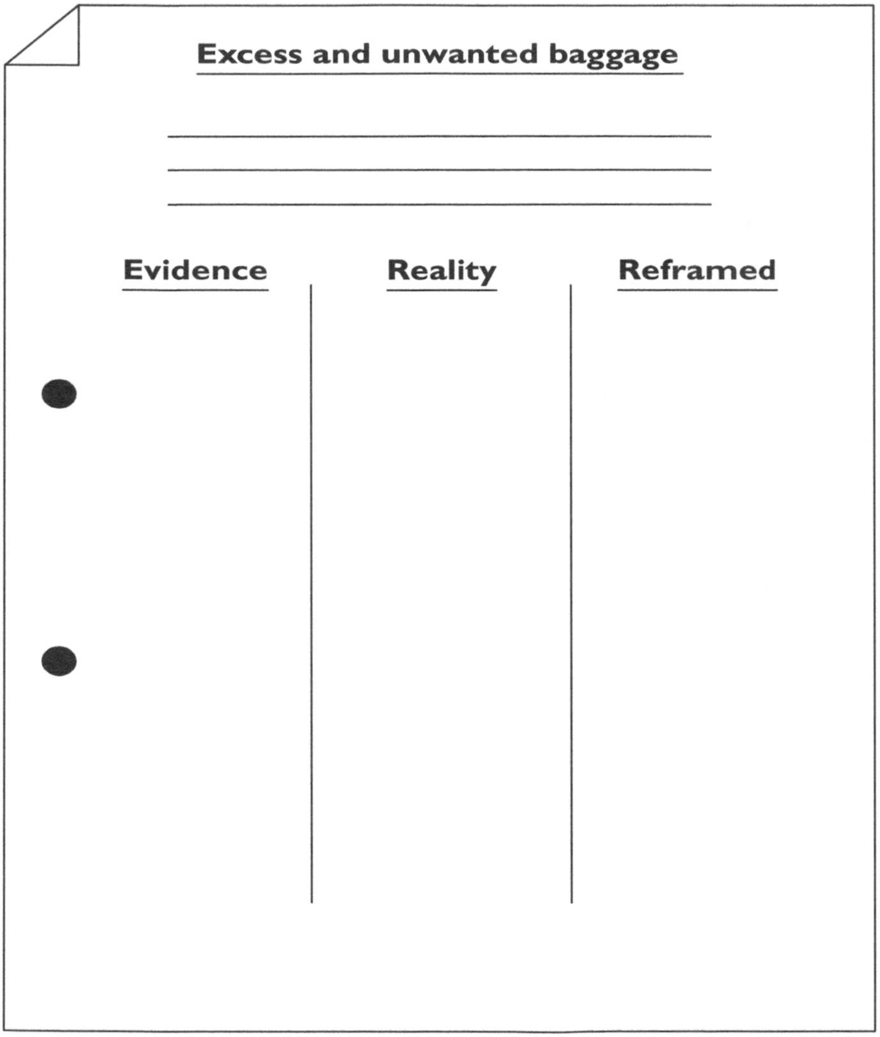

Excess and unwanted baggage

_____

_____

_____

Evidence	**Reality**	**Reframed**
●		
●		

Figure A.1 Excess and unwanted baggage
Break down and reframe unhelpful psychological baggage. See Exercise 2.1.

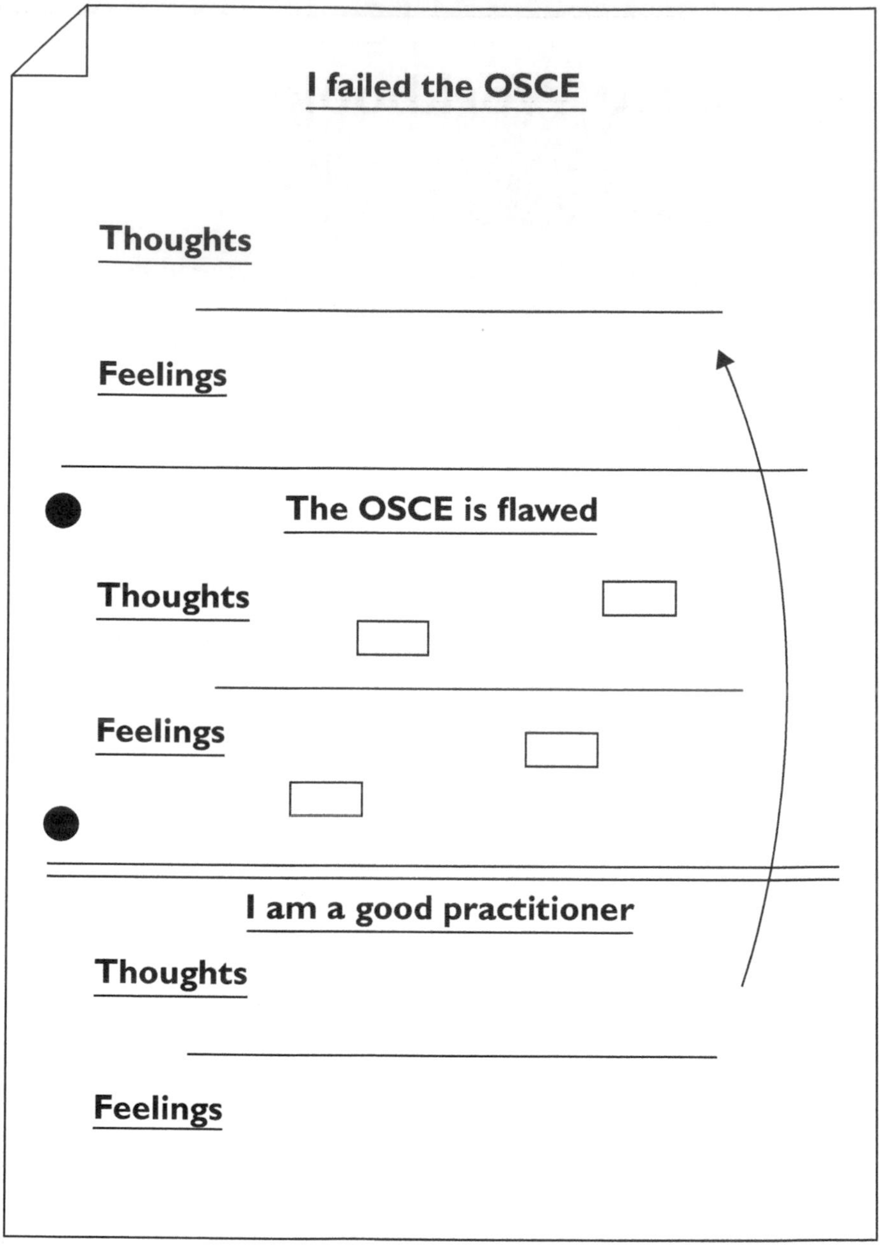

Figure A.2 Challenging your beliefs
Explore and bypass those unhelpful beliefs that resolve the conflict of 'failure' and 'success'. See Exercise 3.1.

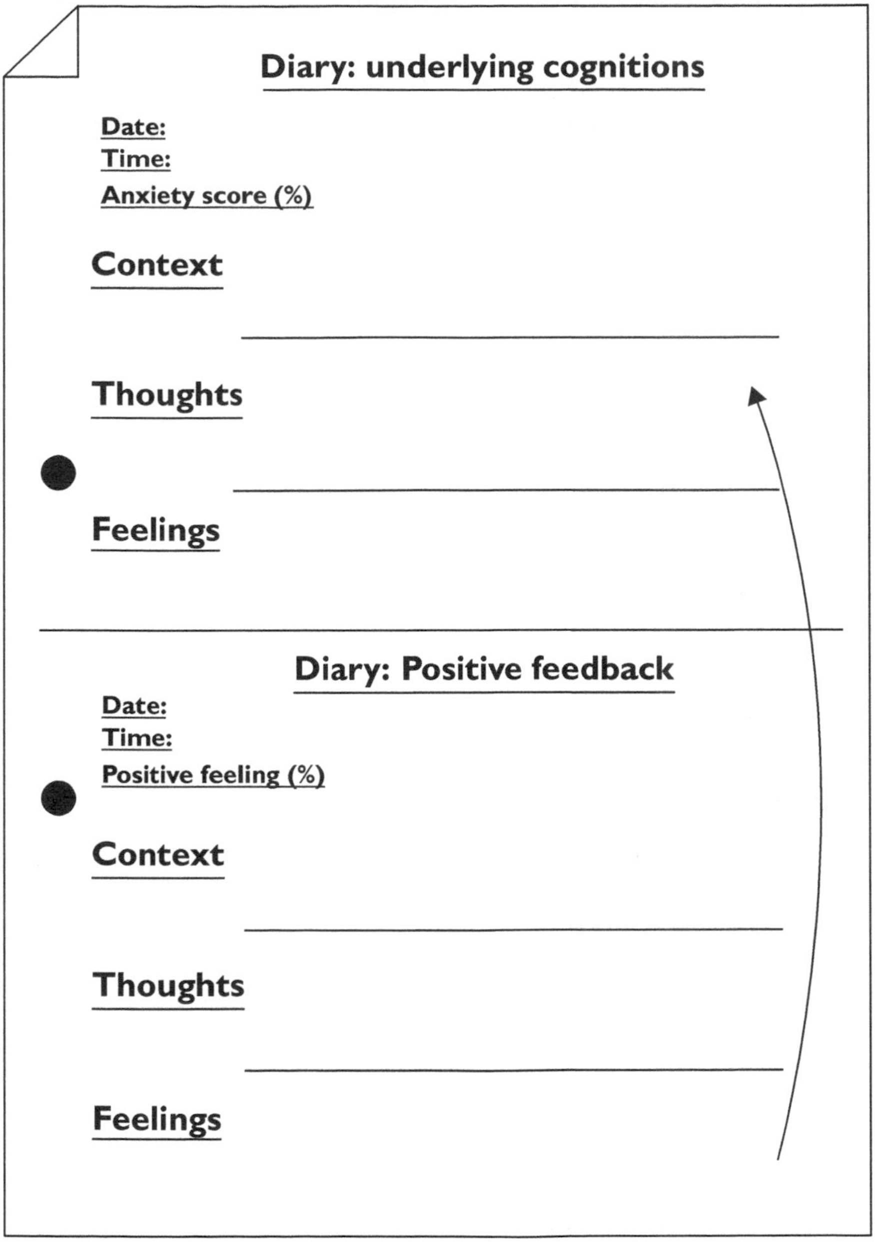

Diary: underlying cognitions

Date:
Time:
Anxiety score (%)

Context

_____

Thoughts

 ● _____

Feelings

Diary: Positive feedback

Date:
Time:
 ● **Positive feeling (%)**

Context

_____

Thoughts

_____

Feelings

Figure A.3 Diary: underlying cognitions
Keep a diary, to identify and monitor those thoughts that make you feel anxious, along with those that are more positive and empowering. Review and explore the nature of your underlying cognitions. See Exercise 4.1.

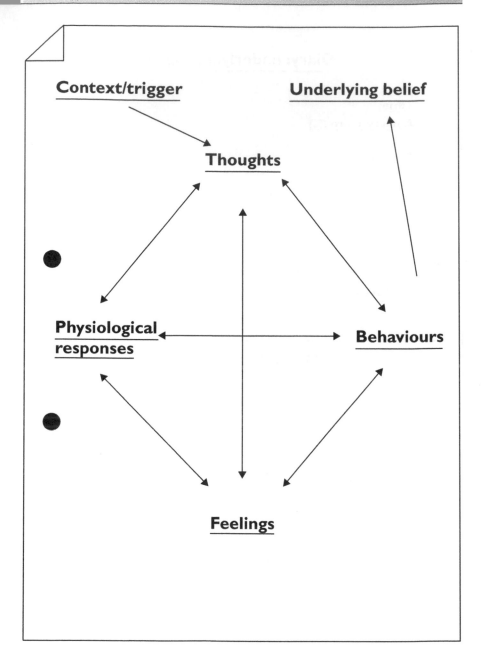

Figure A.4 Breaking the cycle
Identify behaviours that you can modify, in order to disrupt the reinforcement of unhelpful underlying beliefs and cognitive processes. See Exercise 4.2.

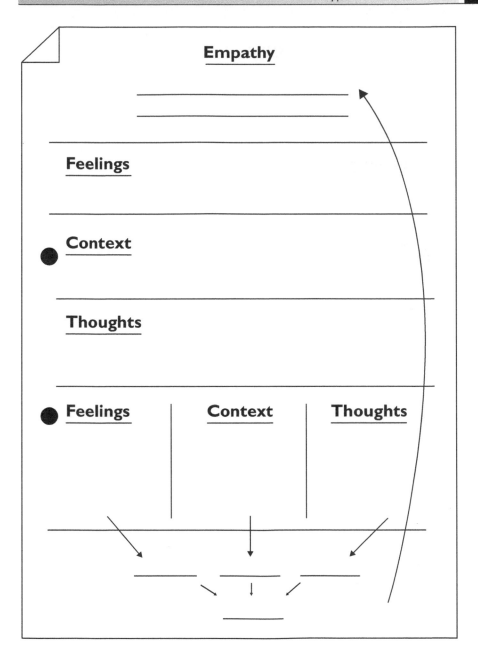

Figure A.5 Dissecting and repackaging empathy
Record, deconstruct, and explore your subjective experience of empathy. Distil the essence of your empathy and develop empathy 'triggers' to employ in your OSCE. See Exercise 7.1.

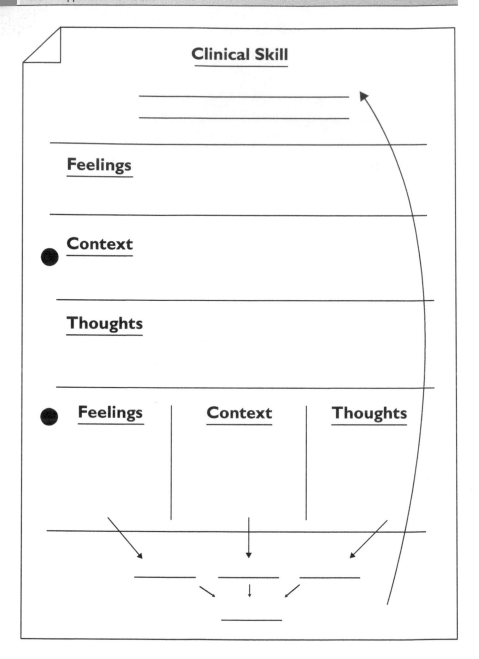

Figure A.6 Dissecting and repackaging clinical skills
Repackage your modular clinical skills by linking them to emotive contextual elements. Deconstruct and distil the essence of these linked modular skills, and develop skill 'triggers' to employ in your OSCE. See Exercise 11.3.

Index